List of Contributors

Asmaa Al-Kadhi

Imran Aslam

Sandhya Chowdary

Noah Z. Feldman

Aleksandra Florek

Farah Moustafa

Jean-Phillip Okhovat

Kelly Quinn

Liz Ramsey

Irma M. Richardson

Brandy H. Sullivan

Acknowledgments

Special thanks go to Joe Jorizzo for his support to the entire research program at Wake Forest since his founding of the Department of Dermatology, Alan Fleischer for his leadership and support of research during his time as chair, Raj Balkrishnan for introducing the MEMS cap into our research to monitor adherence (and all his other invaluable contributions to our understanding of adherence and health care delivery issues), and Amy McMichael for continuing to support the Center for Dermatology Research as the current Department Chair.

We would like to acknowledge all the members of the Center for Dermatology Research who have contributed to our research on adherence, patient satisfaction, and patient behavior over the years, especially our fellows Tamara Housman, Mandeep Kaur, Christie Carroll, Judy Hu, Michael Kucenic, Jennifer Krejci-Manwaring, Mark Tusa, Dan Pearce, Kim Cayce, Chris Yelverton, Sarah Taylor, Brad Yentzer, Jenna O'Neill, Tushar Dabade, Michelle Levender, Cameron West, Cheryl Gustafson, Laura Sandoval, Karen Huang, Arash Taheri, Megan Kinney, Ashley Feneran, Swetha Narahari, Amir Al-Dabagh, Farah Moustafa, Hossein Alinia, and Sara Moradi-Tuchayi; Vishal Khanna; Clinical Studies Director Adele Clark; Project Manager Irma Richardson; our tireless administrative assistant Rachel Starling; and CEO of our commercial partner Causa Research, Robert Anderson.

Dan Ariely has been especially instrumental in getting us interested in behavioral economics, as well as providing us with an inexhaustible supply of research to cite. Richard Thaler, Cass

Sunstein, and Charles Duhigg have also encouraged us to explore this exciting field.

We would like to thank the Association of Psychocutaneous Medicine of North America (APMNA) and European Society for Patient Adherence, Compliance, and Persistence (ESPACOMP) for allowing us to present this research at their annual meetings and giving feedback, particularly Mohammad Jafferany, Rick Fried, Liset van Dijk, Annemiek Linn, Yoleen van Camp, and Betsy Sleath. Special thanks to John Koo.

The Center for Dermatology Research has been funded by Galderma Laboratories, L.P. since 2003. We are very thankful for their support that has enabled us to continue exploring new research directions that will improve patient outcomes.

We thank all the patients who have taught us so much and broadened our understanding about the patient-provider interaction, especially those who have participated in research studies.

We would like to thank our families. Steve Feldman thanks Ed & Fran Feldman for their unceasing support. Scott Davis would like to thank Jim and Jean Davis.

Foreword

Why do we do what we do? How can we effectively influence others to do what we wish them to do for amelioration of their physical and emotional well being? Understanding the underpinnings of these questions and gaining access to succinct and effective answers is the recipe for enhancing the likelihood of success in all facets of our personal and professional lives. This book offers these coveted answers and it should be mandatory core curriculum reading for medical students, residents, and practicing clinicians again and again! The editors of this manuscript are truly a dynamic duo. The brilliance, clinical acumen, effective and affable teaching style, and amazingly prolific contributions to the literature of Steve Feldman MD, Ph.D have been a "wake up call" and "game changer" for clinicians in all nations on our ever interconnected globe. His perspective as a "MD dermatologist" and "Ph.D epidemiologist" offer us a unique scientific and global interpretation of the current state of affairs in medicine and life. His recent book 'Compartments" is a fun adventure of vignettes that thoughtfully encourage us to realize how our opinions and appraisals of others are colored by the limited view afforded by the compartments within which we live and view the world. Scott Davis, MA is an enthusiastic, effective, and finely educated researcher and administrator. He brings to this publication an impressive array of publications especially in the areas of general dermatology, motivation, adherence, and behavioral economics. This book seamlessly brings together recognized experts in human behavior to offer their succinct explanations and recommendations to improve patient adherence and satisfaction. The sad reality is that brilliant grasp and fluency with the literature and superb treatment regimens are essentially useless if they are not confidently and positively embraced by patients. This book is the "how to" handbook to make clinicians more effective in their endeavors to deliver quality care that will be more likely embraced by patients. Read it, re-read it and take a fresh look at yourself and your patients. It will be time well spent. Truly, look at patient blogs and patient ratings of clinician competence and compassion. Understanding them better will make you a more effective and esteemed clinician.

Richard G. Fried, MD, PhD
Dermatologist, Yardley Dermatology
Yardley, Pa.

Table of Contents

Chapter 1
Introduction: What is Behavioral Economics?
Scott A. Davis and Steven R. Feldman

Imagine you are out on a rainy Sunday afternoon with some friends to see the new *Hobbit* movie. As you buy your ticket, the theater's sales clerk says, "Would you like a membership? It is on sale today for $10/year (charged to your credit card, renewing automatically, usual price $25/year) but with your membership you get a FREE popcorn and drink today, which is worth $11, so you actually get $1 back right away. Don't miss this opportunity!" The clerk has already used many behavioral economics principles in this marketing effort. As we will see in this book, she used the "FREE! effect", used anchoring to make you think the popcorn and drink are worth $11, and got you to feel invested in this movie theater (and partially commit to going there in the future) through "membership". She also used a default option by having the membership renew automatically, suggested a credit card to negate the salience of cash, and invoked loss aversion by saying not to miss the opportunity.

This might seem like trickery once you think about how successfully you were manipulated into buying the membership. However, what if these same tactics could be used to "encourage" people into performing positive health behaviors? The idea is not so far-fetched as it may sound. In a perfectly rational world, people would perform every health behavior that is good for them: take all their medications every day, always exercise, always eat right, never smoke, and never hide any information from their doctor. They would also save their money and not be influenced by carefully honed sales pitches and "great deals". In fact, people do not perform these strictly rational behaviors, yet with the benefit of psychological knowledge, we can understand how, when, and why they do not. And just as marketers do not treat the consumer's reluctance to spend money as an insuperable obstacle, we as health care professionals do not need to treat patients' reluctance to perform healthy behaviors as "just the way things are".

Behavioral economics is the study of social, cognitive, and emotional factors that affect human economic decisions. Like many other social scientists in the 19th and early 20th centuries, economists tried to develop the field of economics as a completely objective, scientific field like physics. They tried to form theories that would predict human behavior with mathematical precision. Actually, Heisenberg's uncertainty principle soon showed that even in physics, perfectly predicting the behavior of particles was impossible, but economists did not give up. The epitome of economists' striving toward an objective, scientific ideal was rational choice theory. According to rational choice theory, humans were basically rational actors who would weigh the costs of an action against the benefits, and if the benefits outweighed the costs, they would perform the action. For example, when deciding whether to park illegally, they would weigh the cost C of a parking ticket, the probability P of being ticketed, and the benefit B of parking in the illegal spot rather than finding a legal spot. Then they would park illegally if and only if C*P was less than B.

Eventually, some economists realized that rational choice theory had severe limitations when it came to describing actual human behavior. First, rational choice theorists predicted that people would behave the same way every time, given an identical situation. However, emotional factors often intervened, such as a person being more likely to overeat after going through a situation that demanded extra willpower. Second, rational choice theory suggested that the response to a question would not be influenced by its wording; people would always make the same choice even if a question was framed differently to different groups of people. Third, the theory said people's reaction to a situation would increase proportionally as the probability of the situation increased. In a seminal 1984 article, "Choices, Values, and Frames", Daniel Kahneman and Amos Tversky demonstrated that all these assumptions of rational choice theory were violated so frequently that rational choice theory alone had little value in predicting actual human behavior.[1] Experiments routinely demonstrated that a large majority would make one choice under a certain set of conditions, but the opposite choice when the emotional or social context of the decision changed, although the two sets of choices were mathematically identical.

Behavioral economics rests on the realization that people behave in irrational ways, but the deviations are not random and actually quite predictable. Ironically, long before behavioral economics was a recognized field, experts in marketing had already been exploiting advanced psychological knowledge about their customers for decades. For example, it appears that Alfred Sloan grasped the principle of salience (see Chapter 4) when he directed General Motors to start making annual model changes in the 1920's to outcompete Ford. It took many more years to codify the major principles, some of which are still being debated. The field of behavioral economics applied to health care is still in its infancy, but much interesting research has already been performed.

The premise of this book is that behavioral economics can be applied to many situations that we as health professionals face every day. The healthy behavior is generally the most rational, but many social, cognitive, and emotional factors intervene and persuade patients to do something considerably different. Furthermore, more often than not, patients think they are being rational when they choose not to follow a healthy regimen. Fortunately, in some cases a simple process of causing the patient to look at a situation differently can dramatically change the behavior. In other cases, modifying behavior is more difficult, but there are still techniques we can use. Usually it isn't a question of whether or not patients' decisions will be influenced by context or framing. They *will* be affected. The doctor's choice is whether or not to try to make it the best possible context. For example, we should try to set a default option of starting a medication immediately; otherwise the opposite behavior (i.e. not filling the prescription) becomes the default (see Chapter 6, Default option).

Each chapter in this book begins by defining a specific principle — a cognitive bias, a way in which people tend to deviate from "rational" thinking — that has been defined in behavioral economics. The chapter then lays out the experiments that have demonstrated how people behave as predicted by the principle. We then give everyday examples of the phenomenon, and conclude with practical examples that apply the theory to medicine. Since behavioral economics predicts that you probably have limited willpower, we anticipate you might turn to the tips at the end of the chapter right away, though we hope you won't skip the "journey" to get to the destination! We hope the book serves equally well as a reference book and as a thorough introduction to this fascinating subject.

PART I

Misperception in Context: How Disease and Treatment Look Different Depending on Context

Chapter 2
Anchoring
Imran Aslam, Scott A. Davis, and Steven R. Feldman

Anchoring is a cognitive bias that describes the tendency to use one piece of information (the anchor) as a reference point for determining the value of other items.[2] In rational choice theory, people were assumed to judge the value of goods objectively without being influenced by unrelated reference points, but research in behavioral economics shows that most of the choices and decisions we make can be traced back to a certain anchor. Selecting a logical anchor is the foundation for making sound decisions. In this chapter we will delve into the concept of anchoring and discuss how we select anchors and explore their role in our decision making.

Background and History
In 1974, cognitive psychologists Amos Tversky and Daniel Kahneman collaborated on a series of experiments that demonstrated anchoring and its utility in predicting human errors. In one of their studies, participants were instructed to estimate the percentage of African countries in the United Nations. Prior to giving an estimate, participants were required to spin a wheel numbered from 0-100 and then told to indicate whether that number was higher or lower than the value of the quantity. At the end of the study, researchers found that there was a significant correlation between the number obtained from the wheel and the participant's estimate. The findings of this study demonstrated that an arbitrary value suggested to an individual may

subconsciously evolve into an anchor and result in faulty conclusions.[3]

Another more recent experiment conducted by Ariely, Loewenstein, and Prelec further supported these findings. Ariely and colleagues had students write down the last two digits of their social security number and then asked them to estimate the price of a bottle of wine upon which they would eventually bid. The results of the experiment showed that, surprisingly, students with "highest ending social security numbers bid highest, and students with lowest ending numbers bid lowest."[4] The social security number served as an anchor and affected people's judgments, despite being completely arbitrary (Table 1).

SSN (last 2 digits)	Top 20%	Bottom 20%
Quality of wine noted by individual students	Superior	Superior
Perceived price	$27.91	$8.64

Table 1: Contextual effect of random subconscious factors like Social Security Number (SSN). College students were asked to price a bottle of wine keeping the last two digits of their social security number in mind. Though the students were aware of the quality of the wine, the perception of the actual cost of the wine was influenced by their social security number.

In this experiment social security numbers were used;

however, researchers could have practically proposed any question that would in turn serve as an anchor. Subjects were aware that their social security number had nothing to do with the price of a bottle of wine; yet, somehow thinking about this arbitrary number influenced their price estimates.[4] What is the explanation for this? Tversky and Kahneman proposed that the arbitrary anchor (the social security number) gave participants a starting value which they could adjust to reach a reasonable estimate.[5] Hence even when people are conscious that a certain anchor should have no bearing on their judgment, they are often unable to withstand its influence.[6] As a result they inadequately adjust their assessment away from the anchor. Another explanation proposed by Kahneman is that the mere suggestion of a high/low value can trigger the activation of compatible thoughts of high/low values. For instance if an individual were asked if Gandhi died before or after age 144, and then asked: how old Gandhi was when he died, the mere suggestion of a high number (144) would activate compatible thoughts of high values, and result in a high estimate. Although the age estimate of 144 is obviously wrong, the brain still does not ignore it as rational choice theory would predict.[5]

Examples and Analysis

An anchor can be any idea suggested to an individual. This idea is seeded into an individual's mind and subsequently influences future decisions and behavior, consciously or unconsciously. Commonly, anchors are relevant, unlike the examples above. A consumer intends to purchase a particular used vehicle. He has no idea of the value of the car, so he looks up the manufacturer's suggested retail price (MSRP) and finds it to be $22,000. Now that he has an approximation of how much the car is worth, the consumer starts his search for the used vehicle and decides if a price is too high or too low based on the MSRP he looked up initially. The MSRP in this example is what we refer to as an anchor because it serves as the baseline comparison upon which all future decisions are based. In contrast to the previous section, the MSRP anchor used in this example is relevant and intentionally selected, whereas in Ariely and Tversky's experiments the anchors discussed were neither relevant nor intentional. Anchors can come in all shapes and forms and in the next few paragraphs we will continue to discuss the various applications of anchoring.

We use anchoring on a daily basis to help determine the value of all items big and small, from purchasing a car to our morning cup of coffee. Prior to the arrival of Starbucks, we consumers had an idea or expectation that coffee should be a certain price based on our experience at Dunkin Donuts and other coffee shops. Once Starbucks came along, we were initially shocked by the prices because our anchors told us that Starbucks was expensive. In order for Starbucks to become the successful coffee shop it is today, it had to prove that it was a totally different experience from cheap coffee shops. Starbucks did this by transforming the whole coffee experience into something that was strikingly different than anything customers knew before. From the aroma of freshly roasted coffee beans that strikes us the moment we enter, to the fancy snacks displayed: pecan tart, blueberry scone, to the elaborate names of its drinks like Caramel Brulée Latte, Caffé

Misto, and of course the use of premium coffee beans; Starbucks did everything it could to make itself unique. And in doing so, Starbucks convinced us that our previously held anchors for coffee prices were no longer relevant to Starbucks because Starbucks coffee was different.[4]

When we are deciding how much an item is worth we tend to estimate the value based on the price of products in a similar category, and not on how much pleasure we received from a particular item. One of the reasons for this is because we are anchored by the price of categories. That is, when we consider the price of a cup of coffee we only compare it to other beverages. When we consider the price of software apps we only compare it to other software. What we generally fail to compare is the relative pleasure we get from the app versus the pleasure we get from the coffee. When thinking about software such as apps most of us are very reluctant to spend any money regardless of how nominal the price. The reason for this is because when apps were first introduced, most of them were free. We became anchored to this notion that all apps should be free. As a result we became hesitant to spend even trivial amounts such as $1.00. However, if we changed our anchor and considered how much pleasure we get from a certain $1.00 app and compared that to the pleasure from a $4.00 cup of coffee, we may gain a different perspective on how much an item is actually worth.[7]

Now let us consider an application of anchoring in marketing. Suppose an item is advertised originally at $60.00, but after a 50% price reduction it is now $30.00. A customer might be tempted to purchase this item because he is persuaded that he is getting a bargain. Theoretically though, if the same item were advertised at a price of $30.00, without any price reduction, a customer may be less inclined to purchase it. This phenomenon is another example of anchoring. In the first instance the customer was anchored by the original price and therefore was led to thinking that he was getting a relatively good deal. In the second instance, once the anchor was removed, the relative comparison was no longer made- and the appeal was lost. Retail giants like JC Penney learned this lesson in behavioral economics the hard way. In 2012 sales dropped 25% after JC Penney tried switching their pricing strategy by moving away from coupons and sales to offering a simpler "everyday low price."[8] What the CEO at the time, Ron Johnson, did not understand was that what JC Penney customers wanted more than anything else was the "thrill of getting a great deal, even if it was an illusion." [8] The "everyday low price" approach tried by JC Penney "assumed that customers have some context for how much items should cost. But they don't," according to Alexander Chernev, marketing professor at Northwestern University.[8] Consumers tend to use the original/presale price as the context for determining a good deal. This context is an anchor, and when JC Penney tried removing it, consumers no longer knew how to recognize a bargain and sales plummeted. Once JC Penney realized this, they returned back to their old strategy of coupons and sales in which they marked up the original prices only to mark them back down again in order to give the mirage of a discount.[8]

Another lesson in anchoring can be learned from an airline customer service center. Suppose your 1:00 pm flight is canceled and you need to be in Detroit tomorrow morning. There is an evening flight at 10:00 pm that is open; however, certain reps might say that "the earliest flight available is tomorrow morning," while being fully aware that there is actually a 10:00 pm flight still available. They do this to manipulate the customer's reaction, and they would typically follow up by saying, "but let me see what I can do to put you on an earlier flight which is at 10:00 pm tonight." This is another example of anchoring in which the rep provides a less favorable alternative as an anchor in order to make the other option seem more favorable. Hence, instead of the customer feeling angry at the airlines over his flight being cancelled with a resulting delay, he is now relieved and grateful that the rep helped him fly sooner than he might otherwise have had to do.[9]

Anchoring is essentially a type of mental shortcut that tends to be selected based on convenience and availability (Table 2). The anchor's function is to simplify unknowns in a reasonable time frame. It is a critical aspect of our cognitive process; however, if it is not carefully selected it can lead to irrational conclusions.

Table 2. Common applications of anchoring. The mind easily adopts certain anchors without considering whether they are appropriate, sometimes leading to bad decisions.

Anchor	Examples
50/50 split – A common anchor that the mind tends to adopt automatically	Put 50% in stocks and 50% in bonds. While the optimal allocation actually varies with the saver's age, 50/50 is an easy shortcut Assumption that two possible outcomes are equally likely
Sale prices – "Regular price" serves as an anchor	The sale price seems like a bargain compared to the retail price, but the retail price might have been unreasonably high
Rules of thumb	Engagement ring should be worth 3 months' salary: sets an anchor for comparison. People who spend less or more than the anchor look cheap or generous
Negotiations	The initial offer can influence the rest of the negotiation. High initial price leads to high final price
Accommodations made by customer service centers	Customer service reps deal with angry customers by first saying that there is nothing they can do (setting an anchor of low expectations), and then follow up by offering a small concession, making the consumer feel more grateful instead of angry

Applications in medicine

Anchoring in physicians

Anchoring is a phenomenon that penetrates into all facets of life, including medicine. Physicians, like everyone else, are susceptible to the pitfalls of anchoring; however, in the case of doctors the stakes are much higher. Studies have shown that about 80% of misdiagnoses are the result of cognitive errors such as anchoring.[10] When searching for a diagnosis, it can be very easy to get anchored on all sorts of things; whether it is a first impression, a specific detail in the history, a lab value, or a physical finding.[10] Once the anchor is cast and set, it can become difficult to develop a comprehensive differential diagnosis and easy to ignore new pieces of information that may become available. One example of this relates to an ER physician who had recently made a number of viral pneumonia diagnoses during an epidemic in the community. One of his patients during this time period was a woman who came in with a few signs and symptoms suggestive of pneumonia. However she also had certain critical findings that were inconsistent with pneumonia; such as a negative physical exam, negative chest x-ray, and a negative white blood cell count. Despite these contradictory findings, the ER physician still diagnosed this patient with pneumonia and admitted her to the hospital service. Once the patient was seen by the hospitalist, additional tests and history were obtained, and the hospitalist discovered that the patient had aspirin toxicity. In this example the ER doctor's previous experience with the viral pneumonia epidemic served as an anchor that prevented him from considering other possible diagnoses.[11]

Anchoring in patients

After we diagnose a patient and offer treatment plans the patient always has at least two options: accept treatment or refuse it. Our responsibility is to make sure patients get the best care, and that often times requires us to sell our patients on a certain treatment if we believe it is in their best interest. Some patients require a great deal of convincing and others require little; however, just like any successful salesperson we need to cast resilient anchors. If we understand and utilize anchoring skillfully we can guide our patients to make the right decision in regarding their health. For example, if we tell patients there is "a risk of lymphoma" with TNF inhibitors, some patients will tend to assume it is a 50/50 risk, when it is actually a very small risk. If we describe the risks vaguely, then we may inadvertently set this completely inappropriate anchor. However, if we show them an appropriate graphical display of the magnitude of the risk, they will visualize how unlikely it is.[12] We can also use anchoring to help discourage a patient from an inappropriate treatment by saying "The risk is less than a coin flip," while encouraging a reluctant patient by saying "There is a risk and it is greater than getting hit by lightning." If we skillfully implement anchoring when advising patients we can guide them to better health care decisions. don't describe risks vaguely

In the cosmetic dermatology world, anchoring can be used to establish the risk of complications and adverse outcomes. Cosmetic procedures that have no health benefit to the patient should be considered very carefully. For instance, in a patient that would like to have sclerotherapy, a medical procedure to eliminate varicose veins, we need to clearly emphasize the real risk of scarring, skin color changes and other complications so that the patient understands the possibility of replacing one cosmetic defect (veins) with another (scars).[13] By creating this mental anchor early on, the patient will be better prepared for worst case scenarios and less likely to blame the physician for uncontrollable disappointing outcomes. Cosmetic dermatologists may also want to use anchoring when setting prices to make their services seem like a good deal. Coupons and deals can be implemented to encourage patients to seek treatment. For example, if we ran a one month promotion for 50% off of cryotherapy treatment, we can motivate passive patients to seek treatment for precancerous lesions, skin tags, and other related conditions. However, offering half-price deals through Groupon or Living Social can establish half price as patients' anchor, and may be counterproductive.[14] These half price anchors are troublesome because they will cause patients to consider the discounted price as the new normal, and result in patients delaying treatment until the next promotion. Another problem with half price deals is that they reduce the perceived value of a service, whereas if we do patients a "favor" we can avoid this pitfall. For instance, if we were administering 40 units of botox, we could add another 10 units for free as a "favor" for new patients. This "favor" allows the value of the service to be retained, and it would make patients feel grateful, and help build the foundation for a strong physician-patient relationship. Utilizing this favor approach would elicit a much different reaction from a new patient than say if we were selling 50 units of botox for the price of 40.[14]

Anchoring can also be used in conjunction with positive or negative reinforcement to augment certain health risk behaviors. For example, we can give discounts to patients who quit smoking or lose weight, or we can charge higher rates to patients with high risk health behaviors. This ideology is already observed by many health insurance companies that are known to charge smokers with a higher premium. These are just a few examples of how anchoring can be implemented in the healthcare setting to better serve our patients.

unethical though

Quick Tips

- Use a low anchor to illustrate a low risk, and a high anchor to illustrate a high risk.
- Use a high anchor to set realistic initial expectations for potential problems from cosmetic procedures. Better to under promise and over deliver than to over promise and under deliver.
- Be very careful when offering deals that might set an unreasonably low anchor for the appropriate price for a service.

Chapter 3
Context
Sandhya Chowdary, Scott A. Davis, and Steven R. Feldman

Context is the collection of environmental factors that affect an individual's perception of a given stimulus.

Context allows an individual to make informed decisions by picking up visible and invisible cues from the environment in which they are immersed. Context represents an interplay of spatial and factual information that impacts how events and other stimuli are perceived. Context may be built up in an individual's mind over time using fragments of perceived information and linking these mental contents to each other. [15] Rational Choice Theory assumes that people make decisions based on pre-conceived assumptions of risks and benefits irrespective of context. In other words, Rational Choice Theory assumes that people are well-informed individuals with a tunnel vision mindset of making a choice based on presumed pros and cons. While this presumption may provide good prediction in some situations, it fails in others. [16, 17]

Background & History
Relativism is very similar to contextualism with a few subtle differences. [18] The theory of relativism gained popularity in the ancient world. Around 490-420 BC, Greek philosopher Protagoras advocated relativism saying *"Man is the measure of all things: of the things which are that they are, and of the things which are not, that they are not."*

This was in contrast to the views of other Greek philosophers like Plato and Aristotle. They proposed a theory that truth existed independent of the observer.

The 21st century continues to build upon this theory of contextual thinking patterns. Behavioral economics finds that a person's choices are often malleable and unpredictable, the so called "Tom Sawyer" effect. [19] Though people may have reasonable information to believe that a particular choice may be the right one for them, subconscious context factors make them choose otherwise. As seen in Mark Twain's legendary story, the friends of Tom Sawyer were led to believe that painting a fence was an attractive proposition. These friends surely knew what a hard task painting was but chose to go through with it in the context of Tom's enthusiasm for the task.

Examples and Analysis

The effects of context on perception is seen in certain optical illusions; for example, two circles of the same color may appear very differently when each is presented surrounded by squares of different colors. The effect of context on color perception also explains why veins appear blue even though the blood flowing through them is dark red. The blue appearance of veins is due to the way color is perceived by the human brain. [20] While the vein is actually a pinkish flesh color, it is a bluer shade than the surrounding skin and thus appears blue. Judgments about the personality of people are sometimes based heavily on the context of the environment that surrounds them. For instance, people in the Mid-western region believe that those settled in California are happier due to the favorable weather there. In contrast, the people in California are no happier than their Mid-western neighbors. Similarly, with regards to the climate, a 60 degree Fahrenheit day seems cold in summer and warm in winter.

In the context of taste perception, though cola and ice cream have unique flavors, together, the ice cream makes the cola seem bitter. A person tasting coffee for the first time may enjoy the experience better in a quiet ambience surrounded by the company of good friends rather than in a noisy café.

In the religious context, the concept of reward and punishment is used to influence the actions of people. Attempting to recite or write the Ten Commandments elicited the honest side of people in experimental settings.[21]

The popular air freshener brand of today 'Febreze', failed to make an impression when it was first launched as a product to "kill" bad odors. The people who seemingly needed Febreze the most – those with many pets or other sources of bad odor – were so accustomed to their context that they did not notice the bad smell. Vexed by the unimpressive response of the general public, the manufacturing crew carried out an experiment where they blindfolded some customers. These customers were then led into an area sprayed with Febreze air freshener. All of them agreed there was a refreshing fragrance in the air. When the blindfolds were removed, the customers were shocked to find they were surrounded by dirty laundry and strands of cat fur on the furniture. In the context of being accustomed to a home with moldy smells, customers did not perceive benefit from an air freshener. Rather than emphasizing the need to kill bad odors, the manufacturer thus switched to marketing Febreze as a product that everyone would want to use when they finished cleaning. [22]

In the context of mob mentality, people sometimes do crazy things in a group which they would otherwise refrain from doing if they were alone. For example, mobs instigate feelings of violence and vandalism triggering off a chain reaction among people to act in a similar violent manner; cults paralyze the logical thought process of an individual making them do bizarre, outlandish acts. On the other hand, people in a group may change for the better than if they were on their own. Medical communities, church members and members of community service programs often work together for the betterment of the society that surrounds them.

In the context of Behavioral Economics, customers and retailers follow a "price-image" of a product.[23] This means that a pattern is followed in deciding whether a product is worth a particular price. Customers tend to compare prices within a store rather than with other stores. In order to make an expensive product seem more reasonably priced, retailers tend to do the following:

i.   Horizontal extensions: Adding options in the same price range which differ very slightly but tactically from the product on sale (e.g. a new color).

ii.   Vertical extensions: Decreasing the price image by pairing a low priced product with an upscale product or increasing the price range by doing vice versa. For instance, the sales of a moderately priced bread-maker increased when an even higher priced upscale bread-maker was added to the mail order catalogue.

Applications in Medicine

Context strongly influences the way people view their medication regimens. A hard regimen might seem easy if the previous regimen was harder. Taking a medication daily is difficult, but might seem easy to someone who had been trying to take it twice a day. Spraying a sunscreen might seem more feasible than smearing cream before heading outdoors.

Getting accurate information from patients, particularly regarding their adherence to treatment can be difficult. Based on the Ten Commandments experiment, invoking a religious context by asking the patient about their religious affiliation might help elicit more honest, accurate information on their compliance to medication and other health behaviors. Making the topic of honesty salient (see Chapter 4, Salience) may serve as a subconscious cue that we want honest information, not polite white lies. The religious context may also remind the patient of how they are able to confess mistakes and receive forgiveness and understanding in their place of worship. By invoking this context, we may suggest that our office is a similarly nurturing environment where we do not give patients a tongue-lashing for their poor adherence, but offer encouragement and a helping hand.

Using peer pressure, the context of altruism can improve health behavior. If people fear letting the group down, they will take actions they would not take if no one was watching. For example, Alcoholics Anonymous is the most effective way for alcoholics to give up this vice. The accountability to the members of the group plays a big role for this success. Alcoholics Anonymous also requires members to confess the harm they have done to others as a result of their drinking, neutralizing the perception that alcoholic behavior is only the drinker's own private business. Placing the behavior into a group context can completely change the alcoholic's cognitive process and may cause alcoholics to realize that their behavior is causing them to lose friends.

Similarly, smoking bans became more widely supported once the emphasis was placed on secondhand smoke (harm done by the smoker to others) rather than harm done to self. Decades of surgeon general's warnings about cancer and heart disease risk had little impact, perhaps because smokers felt competent to judge the cost/benefit to themselves, and thought that the pleasure they experienced outweighed the risks. However, a new strategy emphasized the ways that smokers were harming others' health by smoking. For example, people who smoked in restaurants were harming the health of the restaurant employees, who had to breathe carcinogenic air whenever they were on the job. Soon, smokers could see that the majority of people were willing to vote for statewide bans on smoking in restaurants, even in states with a history of "pride in tobacco". Smokers began to feel more peer pressure against their smoking, which led many to feel that their social lives would be better if they quit. Some may have even had the alarming experience of seeing themselves ostracized by their ex-smoker peers, who, unlike lifelong nonsmokers, were not afraid to voice their opinions about how bad smokers smelled.

It may seem like a stretch to exploit the group context in quite the same way for medication adherence, but in some cases, low adherence can do harm to others. Poor adherence to antibiotics accelerates the development of drug-resistant strains of pathogens, which can harm everyone. Adherence to HIV medications is higher in Africa than in the US,[24] probably a consequence of greater interdependence in Africa, where many people may be dependent on an HIV patient. This type of HIV patient may feel they are letting down many family members if they die, which is less often the case for American patients. Thus, for potentially fatal chronic conditions such as hypertension or diabetes, we may want to emphasize the effects on loved ones if the patient were to die or become incapacitated. Even when low adherence does not do harm to others, a support group may still help to normalize the adherent behavior and reinforce positive social norms.

Quick Tips

- Patients assess the difficulty of a treatment regimen in the context of their previous regimens.
- Invoking a religious context may encourage the patient to think about honesty and give more accurate answers.
- A group context can help to highlight the negative effect of a patient's unhealthy behavior on others.

Chapter 4
Salience
Jean-Phillip Okhovat, Scott A. Davis, Asmaa Al-Kadhi, and
Steven R. Feldman

Salience is the quality of standing out relative to other items.
People's senses are much more prone to notice a sight, sound,
or smell that stands out. People also place more weight on
particularly vivid and memorable examples of a specific
phenomenon than more typical examples of the same
phenomenon. Although salience can cause people to make
irrational decisions, it can also have positive effects: we can
help our patients by giving salient examples that might stick
in their memory and influence behavior profoundly.

Background and History
One of the earliest theoretical writings leading to the modern
conception of salience was a 1977 article by Richard Shiffrin
and Walter Schneider.[25] After doing a host of experiments
asking subjects to identify various letters or digits in memory
sets of various sizes and traits, they described how salient
stimuli activate automatic brain reactions, which are more
efficient in most cases than rational thought. For example,
salience ensures that you notice safety threats immediately
and automatically respond accordingly, such as by slamming
on the brakes if you see a stopped car on the highway far
ahead. If you had to think about whether to respond to the
salient stimulus or another one, you might respond too
slowly.

Salience has common effects in day-to-day lives. Consumers

spend less money when required to use cash. Cash is salient; when patients pay with credit cards, the money they spend is less salient, and they spend more.[21, 26] Salience also affects honesty. Golfers cheat more frequently by the less-salient methods of moving the ball with a club or their foot, rather than the more guilt-inducing method of picking up the ball and moving it.[21] The principle that more dishonesty can be expected when salience is reduced is not limited to golfers. White-collar crime, such as backdating stock options, is easier to rationalize than stealing equal amounts of cash.[27] Similarly, but on a lesser scale, people will take pens or borrow a stapler from someone's desk but are less likely to steal cash.

Examples and Analysis
Salience has a major impact on people's thinking. People have a far greater fear of a terrorist attack on an airplane than they do of dying in a car accident, even though the latter is a far more common form of death. The terrorist attack stands out much more in the mind; the more graphic the image is, the greater the impact. Similarly, an earthquake in San Francisco measuring 8 on the Richter scale and causing a major flood may seem more likely than a major flood west of the Mississippi; the latter is of course, more likely, because it includes the possibility of a flood in San Francisco.

The importance of salience can be seen in a recent story about the Tesla Model S electric car. In August 2013, this car was given five stars by the National Highway Traffic Safety Administration in crash test ratings; within two days, the stock of the company increased by 2%.[28] However, on October 1, 2013, a Tesla Model S drove over a metal object, which punctured a hole through a plate protecting the car's battery resulting in a fire; the share price then fell by 10% in the next two days. The single rare adverse event had a far greater impact on perception of the car than the far more important, more generalizable, systematic information on safety. This example demonstrates how salience can have a tremendous and influential impact on people's view of a product. In this example, the car's fire was much more salient than the 5 star crash test ratings and numerous other accolades it received. A special case of salience is negativity bias, where one salient negative event outweighs many positive events (see Chapter 14).

Salience is exploited by salespeople when they suggest using a credit card instead of cash, or paying a large amount in periodic installments rather than a lump sum. Spending cash feels more like spending "real money" in that it is immediately salient that there is less money in our wallet. Behavioral economists call this phenomenon "pain of paying"; cash purchases have much greater salience, and thus induce greater pain of paying, than credit card purchases.[29] For some people, spending money with a credit card feels almost like getting something for nothing, until they get a large bill later and may have to pay interest as well. Memberships that automatically renew (see also Chapter 6, Default option) and get charged monthly to a credit card can be especially insidious. People might join a gym as their New Year's resolution and have the monthly membership fee automatically charged to the credit card. They then quit going to the gym after a few weeks, but keep getting charged. The membership might even be FREE! for the first month, but then the card is charged like clockwork every month thereafter, whereas if people had to pay cash every month, they would feel more pain and might either cancel or make use of the membership.

Salience is used in marketing to increase visibility of brands. Alfred Sloan recognized the power of salience back in the 1920's when he directed General Motors to start making annual model changes to its cars. GM's cars would have some new features each year that allowed the latest model to stand out, making GM owners trend setters. Meanwhile, Henry Ford largely dismissed Sloan's strategy as a fad and did not follow suit until much later. By then, General Motors had taken over first place in the American car market, which Ford would not regain until 2011. Frequent changes in appearance to maximize salience are still a standard tactic, as we can see every time we go to the grocery store with all its "New and Improved!" products. Salient smells are particularly powerful; restaurants in a mall or airport know they must make sure people can smell them from as far away as possible.[30]

Applications in Medicine

The idea of salience can be applied to medicine in a variety of ways. We can put salience to use in encouraging better sun protection by changing how we discuss skin cancer. Telling patients that sunscreen can prevent skin cancer does not have the same salience as telling patients that "sunscreen can help prevent you from developing a golf-ball-sized, ulcerating, odious skin cancer of your nose that requires removal of your nose, leaving a gaping hole in the center of your face, but don't worry, you would be able to wear a nice latex nasal prosthesis to cover the hole". The description of the specific possibility of a golf-ball-sized nasal tumor can have greater impact than the description of skin cancer in general, even though skin cancer in general is far more likely and includes the special case of the golf-ball-sized tumor.

photo of skin cancer too

Salience also influences patients' views of medications. Oral retinoids, such as isotretinoin (Accutane), are used for the treatment of nodulocystic acne. One publicized adverse effect from the use of isotretinoin, a synthetic form of vitamin A, is rare incidence of depression, with suicides having been reported. Although the use of isotretinoin is closely monitored, and the risk of serious depression is rare, the salience of reported suicides may turn off a patient from considering the use of a highly effective drug. Even when the side effects are not so dramatic, they can be more salient than the benefits of the drug. The patient may be accustomed to the suffering from the disease, and by comparison, the drug's side effects seem worse than the disease. For example, many antidepressants cause sexual dysfunction, which may be more salient than the improvement in brain serotonin induced by the antidepressant. Thus, we should anticipate that patients will be concerned by risk of side effects and be sure to put them into proper perspective. If fear of a particular side effect bothers the patient greatly, we can offer to switch them to a different treatment without that highly salient side effect. A greasy ointment that smells bad (highly salient negative properties) may be much less useful than a theoretically less potent less messy vehicle that is easy-to-use.

Salience can be used both to discourage risky health behaviors and to promote healthy behaviors. Many insurers are now offering financial incentives for patients who engage in certain healthy behaviors, such as losing weight. Charging a lower premium may not be salient to patients, most of whom would not notice a small change in their monthly paycheck. Therefore, Loewenstein, Asch, and Volpp suggest that payments rewarding healthy behavior might be paid as separate checks, or patients achieving their goal could be enrolled in a lottery to win a larger amount.[31] Similarly, given the greater salience of cash, people could be required to pay for cigarette purchases with cash rather than credit cards. Conversely, some positive health behaviors, such as taking exercise classes, cost money. To induce higher rates of these behaviors, it would help to minimize the salience of the cost.

The concept of salience can also be used to target therapeutic strategies and adherence to medications. Skin cancer, which usually occurs decades after starting to use tanning beds, may not be salient for young people. Appearance is highly salient, and educational programs built on the negative impact of UV exposure on appearance may be more salient and effective.[32] Further educating patients about melanoma and non-melanoma risk factors and allowing them to see real photos of patients affected will leave an even more tangible picture that will promote better health behaviors.

Quick Tips

- Things that stand out in the mind are noticed much more than those that do not.
- Giving a vivid example of a phenomenon, such as a very large and unsightly tumor for skin cancer, is more effective than a general example.
- Incentives may be much more effective when taking the extra effort to make them more salient.

Chapter 5
Framing
Noah Z. Feldman

Framing is the tendency for a person to change how they value a set of options based on the current frame of reference they are in, or the "frame" from which the option is presented. Many effects constitute framing, and it is wide enough to encompass the Endowment Effect and Loss Aversion (Chapters 15 and 13 respectively); however, we will cover several other examples of framing in this Chapter, including the "Free!", "Ikea", and "Certainty" effects.

The **Free! Effect** occurs when an option's apparent price point is zero, overriding other qualities that affect the choice of the option. For instance a person might choose free water over 25 cent orange juice, even though they would buy the same orange juice for a dollar if the water was 75 cents.

The **Ikea Effect** holds that when someone puts work into obtaining or building something personally, he or she values that thing more highly. The namesake example is that a chair from Ikea (such as the one in which I am currently sitting), which requires assembly when you bring it home, will feel more comfortable and psychically valuable than an otherwise identical chair that was bought preassembled.

The **Certainty Effect** states that people prefer an option with no risk of failure over a risky option with higher payoff, even if the latter is mathematically better. For example, someone might prefer a guaranteed 2% interest government bond over

an equivalent corporate bond with 4% after-tax interest and a
1% failure rate.

Background and History

The **Free! Effect** was described by researcher Dan Ariely after
an experiment involving chocolates.[33] The Researchers set up
a number of stand selling two types of chocolates (Hershey
Kisses and Lindt Truffles) and a sign proclaiming "one per
customer." When participants ("customers") approached the
stands, they were shown one of two price schemes. In one the
truffles were 15 cents and the kisses were a penny, whereas in
the other, the truffles were 14 cents and the kisses were free.
Ariely explains that in both cases participants are making the
decision whether or not to spend 14 cents to upgrade to the
truffles, but the framing of the 14 cent higher costs differs in
the two schemes. To protect against the influence of making
change on the result, the experiment was repeated at the end
of a MIT cafeteria line, where students already had their
wallets out, and the results were essentially equivalent.

Under the 15 cent versus 1 cent scheme, the truffles were
selected 73% of the time. In a rational model this should also
be true for the second scheme. Instead, truffle purchases
plummeted to 31% when priced at 14 cents and the kisses next
to them were free. Ariely puts forward two explanations for
this. The first posits that the idea of "free" holds emotional
impetus for us; there is some pride or joy or pleasure in
getting to say that the chocolate we're eating was garnered for
nothing but a word. The other theory is that when we see that
something is free in the monetary sense, we ignore the other
costs of consuming it (calories, not getting a Truffle, time etc.)

because we've already heard that it is free. There is one last theory, but it will be discussed at the end of the Examples and Analysis section.

The **Ikea Effect** is a very recent idea that has its roots in the increasing popularity of items, normally manufactured en mass, that are being sold as do-it-yourself projects: Legos, paint-and-print-t-shirts, and, most distinctly, Ikea furniture, just to name a few.[34] The most significant study on this effect split subjects into two groups. One group was asked to review a premade Lego car while another was asked build a Lego car based on a very stringent set of instructions (so that the cars would be identical to those of the control group). Then, both groups were asked how much they would be willing to spend to buy the car. Those that made the car themselves were willing to pay more than twice as much for the same colorful plastic blocks as those who were not emotionally attached to the cars.

There are, again, two basic explanations for the Ikea Effect. The first revolves around competence: people are intrinsically confident in their abilities, so they trust the quality of something they themselves build over something that arrives all nice and pre-packaged on their doorstep. There is also a bit of cognitive dissonance going on in this view of confidence. When thinking about whether something is that they've made is worthwhile, people are forced to ask themselves if they are good at building things. If they were to give a low price for the car, that would mean the answer is no; this causes people to inflate the price they are willing to pay. This theory was further defended in variations of the experiment where subjects were required to rapidly do a series of simple yet frustrating math problems (lowering their sense of competence) before being asked their price: these cases had even greater evidence of the Ikea effect than before.

The **Certainty Effect** was first found in a French study, where two groups of participants were asked to consider 2 sets of two bets, and for each set, choose between the two bet options.[35] Look at Group 1 in Table 1 and think about which of those two gambles you would prefer to take. In the experiment, overwhelmingly people tend to prefer gamble A. When people are presented the two gamble options in Group 2, they tend to prefer gamble B. Both of these choices make sense on their own, but they are inconsistent when taken together. Based on probability, option B is significantly better in both cases (10% of 500 is 50, 11% of 100 is 11). The group you're in shouldn't affect your choice, however; switching from group 1 to 2 simply involves turning 89 chances at $100 into 89 chances at none. This result is commonly explained through the idea that people prefer to be certain in their future, even when that means picking a gamble that is mathematically weaker. When certainty is shorn from their grip however, people will go for the mathematically "correct" option.

Group 1				Group 2			
Gamble 1A		Gamble 1B		Gamble 2A		Gamble 2B	
W	Chance	W	Chance	W	Chance	W	Chance
		$100	89%				
$100	100%	None	1%	None	89%	None	90%
		$500	10%	$100	11%	$500	10%

(W=Winnings)

Table 1. Certainty Effect. In both cases, Gamble B is mathematically superior. However, in Group 1, Gamble B has a 1% probability of winning nothing, an uncertainty that people tend to place excessive weight on. Thus some people in Group 1 choose A instead.

Examples and Analysis
The **Free! Effect** pops up quite often in everyday life. Public schooling is a major example, as it offers a cost-free alternative to private schooling, though this may be a weak example because the actual cost difference is usually a yawning chasm. The tendency to overeat at an all-you-can-eat buffet restaurant may be a manifestation of the effect. The choice to do

housework oneself, when it could be done by an affordable cleaning service and at the expense of time that could have been used earning wages, is another example.

The housework anomaly can also be explained by the **Ikea effect**, in that people have a predisposition to believe that they are personally competent with housework, even above the competence of those who do it as an occupation. I'm writing this in the holiday season, so let's make some festive examples out of common suburban propensities: homemade turkey feasts, hand-crafted holiday cards, home baked pastries, personally planned and prepared packages of presents; all of these things easily purchased outside of the home, probably both less costly and potentially of higher quality. The Ikea effect becomes more potent as the object constructed required more effort, and less impactful if the object is seen as a failure (I would not value my chair at all if it was still just a pile of parts on the ground, though I may still treasure some of the pottery I made in grade school despite the fact that, objectively, the quality of that pottery would never make a juried exhibition).

The **Certainty Effect** makes for a good explanation of why people buy different types of insurance, even though they are often mathematically inferior to casino betting (if you question that they are at all related, realize that both offer infrequent payoffs that are mathematically inferior to banking the cost of the gamble). By buying insurance, a person flattens his expectations curve so that he has certainty: always having a house and an income minus $100 a month is psychologically more comforting than having a house, an income 99.95% of the time and a 0.05% chance of losing everything, even if the latter option is mathematically "superior."

Astute readers may have noticed similarities between the Certainty and Free! effects. They arise at similar times, and they both result in movement towards "perfect" options (free or certain). One explanation for this similarity is that these are both aversions to the risk of making the wrong decision. This explanation goes as such: when we are deciding which item to buy, we build an estimated curve for the likely value of each product to us. Whichever object has a higher average net benefit minus average cost is the one that we purchase (assuming we must choose exactly one). Thus the free item has a 100% chance of at least some benefit, making the certainty effect kick in and increase the preference for the free item.

Applications in Medicine

Often patients may have the choice of a new, improved brand name drug versus a less costly generic alternative. If the generic is free, they may be likely to choose it over a brand name drug whose choice would require a copayment; if both drugs were to have copayments, patients would be more likely to consider the potential benefit that a new, but more expensive drug has to offer. Thus, patients may opt for a somewhat worse treatment for free over a superior treatment for a $25 copayment, yet opt for the better treatment if the copayments on the generic and brand were $10 and $35, respectively. It has become common for pharmaceutical companies to offer coupons that pay part or all of the cost of the co-payment associated with medicines. As well as circumventing market forces (which the co-payment is in place to enforce), the **Free! Effect** may create a considerable incentive to select the brand name medicine if the copayment is fully covered by the coupon. The Free! Effect can also influence people to prefer home remedies or herbal solutions; when people believe that "all natural" products are free of side effects, those products many be chosen over drugs even when those "all natural" products have no proven efficacy.

The Ikea effect also may promote use of home remedies; patients may feel attached to the home remedies in which they have a personal investment. The Ikea effect can also be put to use to increase medication use. When patients are involved with their treatment, when they are making choices and helping to solve problems, when they feel that they are part of their own success, they will predict better outcomes, feel better about the experience in general, and be more invested in the adventure that is regaining their health. To spur this sort of involvement, doctors have a number of strategies: they can educate patients about the options and involve the patient in the choice of therapy; doctors can ask patients to come up with a number of options to help them remember to take their medicine, even if none of the options work particularly well, the process will increase involvement. The Ikea effect results in patients feeling more involved when they make their own decision for which drug to take; if they actively researched the decision and personally went through the process, they will be more involved. Being more involved will not only increase medicine use, but it can also create a placebo effect, in that patients who expect better outcomes generally do better.

The certainty effect is very potent in how it drives behavior, so with great power comes great risk, and doctors should be careful when they say things like, "This procedure always works," or "This medication never fails." These sorts of statements make it very difficult to select the riskier option, even if the other option offers other benefits such as far greater efficacy or lower costs. On the other hand, patients often have trouble distinguishing between 1% and 0.001% risk; saying that the latter has 99.999% success rate instead of a 0.001% risk can help people make the mathematically correct decision.

Quick Tips

- Free! is a special price that strongly encourages patients to choose an option presented as "free".
- As with Ikea furniture, patients who feel personally invested in a treatment are more likely to use it.
- According to the certainty effect, presenting an option as having no risk leads to a much more favorable view of that option.

Chapter 6
Default Option
Kelly Quinn, Asmaa Al-Kadhi, and Steven R. Feldman

The **default option** is a predetermined choice that is provided to an individual to encourage him or her to select an option that, without the default, would require independent decision-making. While not a psychological bias in the traditional sense, the default option has often been implemented to guide consumer decisions. When a choice is offered, the person making the choice can be forced to choose among all the available options with or without giving them a default option that will be used if they do not make a choice. By providing a default option to an individual making an active decision, people's choices can be directed, as people have a tendency to defer to the default, especially when making an alternative choice is complicated and difficult. The use of default options has an extensive history of use and experiment among a variety of situations, including retirement plans, social security, mortgage rates, and even organ donation.

Individuals, when faced with a complex decision with many different choices, will not act in a rational vacuum, but rather will be influenced by their desire for familiarity and ease.[36] And so providing a default option guides decision-making because individuals tend to accept that default option. Similarly, there is a strong tendency not to choose to "opt out" when the default option is to "opt in." This observation is also supported by another behavioral bias that has been described as "the power of inertia," asserting that individuals simply prefer inaction over action regarding decision-making.[36]

Background and History

The default option is a poignant example of the operation of behavioral economics.[37] The most extensively analyzed operation of the default option has been conducted with regard to individual employees and their participation in employer-sponsored defined contribution retirement plans. Employees are more likely to participate in a particular plan if the default option is to participate than if participation requires an active decision to do so. While not a conscientious decision-making tool in classic psychological bias form, having a 'default option' often allows companies to guide their employees or customers and encourage participation in preset plans.

The sentinel study of the default option was carried out by Madrian and Shea in 2001.[38] The pair conducted a two-year analysis of employee behavior at a large Fortune 500 company regarding enrollment in a 401k retirement fund. They studied enrollment behavior between employees who were hired without automatic enrollment in the retirement plan (i.e., had to opt in to participate in the retirement plan) and those who were automatically enrolled (i.e., had to actively opt out of enrollment in the retirement plan). Additionally, they looked at the percentage contribution rate and the selection of investment fund options with defaulted selections versus non-defaulted selections.

Overall enrollment was significantly higher in the group of

employees who were hired after automatic enrollment was implemented. Further, they found that the contribution rate and percent of allocation to the defaulted investment funds remained at the default rate originally set. The tendency to choose the default option violates the expectations of rational decision-making (as a rational decision-maker would make choices based on their economic value regardless of whether they are the default or not) and provides a powerful means to "gently" encourage people to make desired choices.

Examples and Analysis

The default option is appealing to the consumer for a number of reasons. The appeal is most apparent in a situation where the consumer is unfamiliar with the options being presented. As options become more numerous and consequently more confusing, the consumer becomes even less likely to feel comfortable making a decision[5]. It may be intuitive to think that this particular consumer simply chooses the least complex option, but research shows that instead the consumer makes no active decision and yields to the default.

Another reason that a default option is appealing to consumers is because there may exist an inadvertent assumption that it is the option that is in his or her best interest, whether it actually is or is not. In this way, the consumer interprets the default option as advice, even though it does not necessarily serve as such. Regardless of truth, it is one reason that the default option is successful at increasing consumer participation.

Applications in Medicine

The operation of default option behavior is illustrated clearly with population choices regarding organ donation. Organ donation behavior has been widely studied including the impact of how legislation has affected individual organ donation choice. A particularly poignant example is provided by Michielsen in a 1996 publication regarding kidney donation in Belgium.[39] Individuals did not act as classical economics would predict (donate if they wished to donate and refrain if they wished to not donate) but rather made decisions that reflected the default option provided. After implementing a default option of organ donation, the donor rate for kidney donation rose by 86% within two years. Their research also included a direct comparison of donation rates for specific organs between European countries with the default option of donation and those that required informed consent. The rate of donation in countries with default donation was 65% higher for kidneys, 71% for lungs, 100% for pancreas, 110% for livers, and 145% for hearts.

ethical?

Within the practice of medicine, the potential for default options to be used is common. Consider psoriasis, a common skin condition, that has many management and treatment options. Treatment can include a variety of topical agents, forms of phototherapy, several oral options and different injectable biologic agents. Biologics, while very safe and effective, are largely unfamiliar to many patients, which may lead to resistance from patients regarding their use. However, if a particular biologic is presented by the physician as the default option for treatment of severe disease, the patient may be more inclined to accept this treatment option, especially if offered numerous other options described in excruciating detail (which makes just taking the default option an even easier decision).

Is it ethical for physicians to use this type of "nudge" to encourage patients to choose a particular treatment? Assuming the physician feels the recommended treatment is the best option for the patient, then using a default option may be appropriate. Not providing a default option has downsides; there can be so many options to choose from that most patients would be quickly overwhelmed if the decision were entirely theirs; the resulting default may be not to choose any treatment at all, leaving them suffering with untreated disease. Even when offering a default option, the patient has the right to choose a different treatment or to refuse treatment altogether, drawing a parallel with "opting out" of a particular automatic enrollment plan.

This is but one example of the default option in medicine. Many exist and can be helpful when multiple treatment choices exist for a patient. It should be recognized, however, that providing a default option introduces a subtle bias designed to ease the decision-making process and guide individuals to make the choice deemed most appropriate by the one selecting the default.

Quick Tips

- Presenting one treatment as a default option strongly encourages patients to accept that option.
- To increase frequency of a choice, like organ donation or a particular treatment, set the desired option as a default and have people opt out if they prefer not to participate.
- Presenting a large number of other complicated options increases the probability that a patient will choose the default.

Chapter 7
Mental Accounting
Farah Moustafa, Scott A. Davis, Steven R. Feldman

Mental accounting is the concept that consumers create separate mental compartments into which they allocate portions of their money. Money is categorized subjectively-divided by source and/or intent for use. The separation of money into separate "accounts" such as vacation, healthcare, entertainment, etc. affects how the consumer spends his/her money.

Background and History
Mental accounting was described by Richard Thaler, a behavioral economist at the University of Chicago, in 1980.[40] In order to demonstrate his theory of mental accounting, he conducted a survey in which he presented the following scenario:
Imagine that you have decided to see a movie and have paid the admission price of $10 per ticket. As you enter the theater, you discover that you have lost the ticket. The seat was not marked, and the ticket cannot be recovered. Would you pay $10 for another ticket?

He then presented participants with a similar scenario:
Imagine that you have decided to see a movie where admission is $10 per ticket. As you enter the theater, you discover that you have lost a $10 bill. Would you still pay $10 for a ticket to the movie?

In the first scenario, only 46% of survey responders said they would purchase a second ticket. Interestingly, in the second scenario, an almost double 88% said they would purchase the movie ticket. Although the loss of value was the same in both scenarios - $10 – there was a remarkable difference in the consumer response.[41] Thaler describes this behavior of consumer spending as "mental accounting."

Despite both individuals in Thaler' s survey experiencing a net loss of $10, the theory of mental accounting suggests that these two individuals will respond differently to the situation because of their mental compartmentalization of finances. In the first scenario, the individual has already purchased $10 for a movie ticket. Purchasing the ticket is subconsciously accounted for in the consumer's "movie" account. According to Thaler's theory, the reason only 46% of consumers would purchase a second ticket is because the consumer's "movie" account would now be down $20 instead of $10. Because the money is coming from the same mental account, it makes the movie seem too expensive.

In the second scenario however, the ten dollars was lost prior to purchasing the movie ticket. This money was not assigned to the mental account of the "movie," making it easier for the consumer to spend $10 for a ticket.

Examples and Analysis
Mental accounting is much like the financial accounting that occurs within companies. The term "accounting" is defined in Webster dictionary as "the system of recording and summarizing business and financial transactions and analyzing, verifying, and reporting the results". Thaler postulates that we subconsciously make in-the-moment financial decisions based on our preconceived constructs that

make it easier for us to manage our money.

A similar mechanism may explain the behavior of physicians who attended a Psoriasis Education Meeting for Continuing Medical Education (CME). Although the event cost had been completely covered by the sponsors, the CME officer had strongly advised charging a fee for physician attendees. The CME officer said that turnouts for the lectures were always better when there was a fee. A small registration fee of $15 was agreed on for attendance of the lectures. Sure enough, despite severe weather and an ice storm the day before, lecture attendance was nearly perfect. The conference room was filled with physicians who had traveled to Winston-Salem from nearby towns and several states away. What gives? Would attendance have been as good if attendees could register at the event instead of in advance? Probably not. This was a financially secure group of professionals who likely deem $15 an inconsequential amount in the context of their overall wealth. However, the money paid in advance for the lecture was accounted for similar to Thaler's example of the purchased movie ticket. Irrespective of amount, it seems wasteful to not take advantage of that money.

Another use of this phenomenon is in the area of encouraging saving. Many people who don't save money in other situations *will* save a tax refund. A tax refund is a kind of windfall that is not set aside for a specific purpose by many people, and thus might circumvent the mental accounting problem. In their book, *Nudge*, the authors talk about how rational choice theory suggests people should adjust their tax withholding so that they get no refund, but actual humans often like keeping things set up in such a way as to get a refund every year; doing so creates a sense of "free money" in a mental account. [30]

Applications in Medicine

Mental accounting has applications in medicine as well. Consider the patients who have the latest and greatest in electronic devices (smart phones, plasma TV's, etc) but are hesitant about spending money for medications. A common frustration for physicians is the tendency for smokers to spend $4 on a pack of cigarettes *daily* and not to fill a prescription for a month supply of medication for the same price. Part of this phenomenon is due to tobacco addiction. Perhaps, though, part of the issue here is they have "accounted" for daily spending on the unhealthy habit, but are not factoring in a "mental account" that appropriately fits their healthcare needs, however big or small. If the patient is willing, perhaps it would be a good idea to suggest creating a jar or envelope to turn the "mental account" of paying for medications a more concrete physical account in which they can see the dollars adding up. This was supported by a 2013 study out of Yale University that suggested that placing greater emphasis on financial gains of smoking cessation was more effective at cultivating interest in smokers to quit than emphasis of health driven outcomes.[42] Anecdotally, I have seen patients become more motivated when their physicians make this suggestion and even go as far as calculating how much money they can save with smoking cessation over the period of a month, year, etc.

Similar to the above example of pre-paid conference registration fees, it may be feasible to have a pre-pay system for office visit copays to reduce no show rates. It will incentivize patients to make their appointments as they would hate to waste money that has already been "accounted" for in their healthcare spending.

In terms of harnessing money gained from tax returns, we could perhaps persuade people to take part of their next tax refund and put it in a special account to use for improving their health. Thus, a tax refund may be a source of money outside of someone's mental accounts, allowing it to be reallocated to health spending with minimal pain.

Another common problem in the clinical setting is patients being reluctant to fill prescription medications. Separate mental accounts may explain why some patients are willing to pay $10 for an over-the-counter medication, but hate the idea of paying $10 for a more effective prescription treatment because they think it should be fully covered by insurance. While grocery shopping, adding over-the-counter medications can get lumped into the "grocery" mental account, making money for these medications easier for the patient to spend. The patient/consumer may not spend money regularly on prescription medications, if at all. If a patient doesn't even have a mental account for prescription drugs (say, prescription cough meds) because they don't usually buy them, they may feel very reluctant to spend money on the medicine. The mental account of "prescription medications" is not present in the mind of the consumer, so spending any amount of money on these prescriptions seems excessive. For these patients, we could emphasize that since they are going to pay for health insurance anyway, they can then get a $50 treatment for $10 with their insurance. If they paid $10 for an OTC medication, they would only get $10 worth of value. However, by using their insurance to their advantage, they can get a $50 value for $10.

Quick Tips

- People who pre-pay for an expense, such as a conference registration fee or pre-paid doctor visit, are strongly motivated not to lose the amount spent.
- Patients who do not have a mental account for a certain type of healthcare spending may be especially reluctant to spend money on prescription medications.
- Most people perceive a tax refund as a windfall and might be open to spending it on their health.

Chapter 8
Decoy Effect
Scott A. Davis, Asmaa Al-Kadhi, and Steven R. Feldman

The **decoy effect** is the change in people's preference between two items when adding a third choice that is superior to one of the first two options in one property but inferior to both options in another property. In the decoy effect, the choice between two items is influenced by the presence of a third item, which may not have any real relevance to the original decision.

In marketing, this cognitive bias is commonly used to manipulate the consumer into choosing a specific product. As with anchoring (see chapter 2), where a totally irrelevant anchor can be introduced, the consumer struggles to exclude the potentially irrelevant information from the decision making process.

Background and History
The decoy effect was described by Joel Huber, John Payne, and Christopher Puto in 1982.[43] Their experiment involved 153 business students who chose between a target and a competitor with or without a decoy, which was a choice asymmetrically dominated by the target (as described below). Subjects made choices among cars, restaurants, beers, lotteries, film, and television sets. Later, a subset of subjects who had previously made the choice with the decoy repeated the test without the decoy present. The results showed that the decoy did influence preferences, violating the assumption of rational choice theory that the choice between target and competitor

should be independent of the decoy's presence.

Examples and Analysis

The decoy effect is observed when there are two options, such as a lower-priced, lower-quality option A, and a higher-priced, higher-quality option B. For example, A could be a laptop with 8 GB RAM for a price of $500, while B is another laptop with 16 GB RAM and a price of $800 (Table 1). If a "decoy" option C is introduced that is more expensive than both, but intermediate in quality (say, 12 GB RAM and priced at $1000), B will dominate C on both price and quality, increasing sales of B at the expense of A (Figure 1). C may not sell at all, but if the goal is to increase sales of B instead of A, the presence of C helps make B look better and sell more. If the seller prefers to increase sales of A instead, it can introduce an option that is dominated by A but not by B. This option (D) should be lower in quality than both A and B, but intermediate in price (6 GB of RAM for $600). While the attributes are frequently price and quality, they may also be other properties such as convenience or safety.

	A	B	C	D
Amount of RAM (GB)	8	16	12	6
Price	$500	$800	$1000	$600

Table 1. Example of decoy effect with laptops. C is asymmetrically dominated by B but not by A, while D is asymmetrically dominated by A but not by B. The presence of C in the choice set increases sales of B at the expense of A, whereas the presence of D does the opposite.

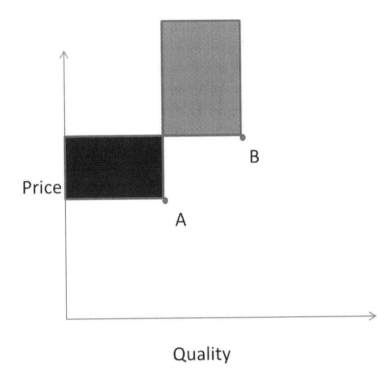

Quality

Figure 1. A decoy C located in the gray region is dominated (better on both attributes) by B but not by A, increasing sales of B. A decoy D located in the black region is dominated by A but not by B, increasing sales of A.

Most of the research on human choice behavior has been confined to the two-alternative case, although most natural situations offer several alternatives (e.g., consumers' choices).[44] An example of the decoy effect with multiple variables occurred recently when one of the authors had a cracked windshield on a car. Several different auto repair shops offered various options for the repair. Company A offered to repair the windshield for $260 with a 1-year warranty, with 2 hours working time and the car ready in 4 hours. Company B offered a price of $280 with a 1-year warranty, coming to the customer's house in 24 hours, with 2 hours working time. Company C offered a price of $260 with a 6-month warranty, with 2 hours working time and ready in 4 hours, and was located 18 miles away. In this case, offer C was asymmetrically dominated by A on the warranty and the travel distance, and had the same price, causing A to look more attractive. The more expensive offer B, though even more convenient than A, did not seem as attractive when C was an option.

If the consumer is assumed to be rational, the choice between A and B should not depend on the presence of other options in the choice set. Either the added quality provided by B should be worth the price differential relative to A, or it should not – independent of whether other options exist. However, the brain fails at being completely rational in this case, and tends to factor in all advertised options, including those that are not seriously considered.

Applications in Medicine

In medicine, decoy effects are not necessarily created intentionally, but can be generated when a new drug or service comes onto the market. For example, treatment options for severe psoriasis used to include primarily just methotrexate or phototherapy. Methotrexate is very convenient in requiring taking only a few pills once weekly, while office-based phototherapy can be very cumbersome to access, but is inexpensive and has fewer side effects. In 2002, biologics were first approved for psoriasis and added to the choice set (Figure 2). Biologics normally have to be self-injected, which is less convenient than a pill, but more convenient than driving to the dermatologist's office multiple times per week. Biologics are also the most costly of the three treatments. Methotrexate dominates biologics on both convenience and cost, while phototherapy does not. Thus the decoy effect may have contributed to continuing declines in use of phototherapy.

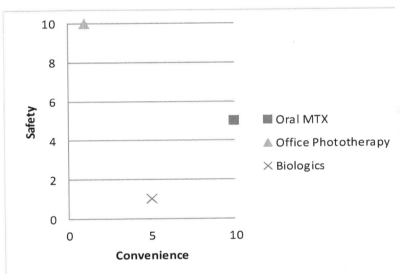

Figure 2. Adding the decoy (biologics), which is more expensive than both original alternatives and intermediate in convenience, increases preference for the alternative (methotrexate) that dominates the decoy.

If clinicians want to steer patients toward choosing a particular treatment alternative over another, mentioning a third alternative that is dominated by the desired alternative may be helpful. High cost is a major problem in the healthcare system. If decoys could be used to increase preferences for cheaper alternatives, fewer people might choose the most expensive treatments. Unfortunately, treatments that would serve as decoys often get removed from the market because there is no reason for anyone to prefer them.

Providers of cosmetic services have a great deal of latitude in offering different packages of services. A decoy effect could be used to direct patients to choose a particular option: offering a high-end package that is dominated by a moderately priced option would increase the perceived attractiveness of the moderately priced procedures over less expensive, less intensive packages.

Some may argue that intentionally manipulating the patient's choice with decoys is unethical. However, the decoy would probably only sway people who do not have any reason to strongly prefer one alternative over the other. It would be an example of a "nudge" to do something beneficial to society that the patient is already willing to do.[30]

Quick Tips

- Decoys can make one option look better relative to another, when one of the options is clearly inferior to the decoy.
- Adding new treatments to the choice set, or removing old ones, can cause irrational shifts in preferences among other options.
- To shift preferences toward a more expensive option, add an even more expensive option; to shift preferences toward a cheaper option, add an even cheaper option.

Chapter 9
Halo Effect
Scott A. Davis, Asmaa Al-Kadhi, and Steven R. Feldman

The **halo effect** is the tendency for one attribute of a person or item to "spill over" and affect perceptions of other attributes of the person or item. Studies have investigated the role of halo effects in the way people treat each other, especially based on attractiveness. Attractive people get rated more highly in unrelated personality traits, are given better grades than unattractive people of the same intelligence, and get treated more leniently by the judicial system.

Background and History
The halo effect was identified by Edward Thorndike in 1920. Thorndike analyzed the ratings made by supervisors on aviation cadets' physical qualities, intelligence, leadership, and character.[45] He showed that observers' estimates of different qualities of the same person tended to be very highly correlated, whereas in actuality, most people would be above average on some traits and below average on others.[45] Also, intelligence should have showed a much stronger correlation with leadership or with character than with physical qualities, but in the ratings, intelligence was about equally correlated with each of the other traits. The raters were instructed very explicitly not to let their opinions of one quality influence their ratings of another, but the correlations showed they could not separately evaluated different qualities as they were tasked to do.

Thorndike's work showed that a "halo" emanating from some

prominent positive qualities of a person, especially attractiveness, affected perceptions of that person in other, even unrelated, areas. Common examples are that attractive people are judged to be higher in intelligence, trustworthiness, happiness, and other positive characteristics than they actually are. Unattractive people are rated lower in the same characteristics than they truly are. Because of these effects, juries will treat an attractive defendant more leniently, imparting bias to the judicial system.[46] Teachers who treat unattractive students unfavorably may create a self-fulfilling prophecy where some students do not get enough positive attention, and develop a negative attitude toward school and learning. A kind, accomplished physician with great patient reviews, loved by residents, and internationally renowned for research might suffer significant damage to his or her reputation if revealed to have HIV infection or some other stigmatizing condition. Halo effects can lead to harmful bias, favoritism, discrimination, and injustice.

Examples and Analysis

Intentional use of the halo effect is most commonly observed when a company strives to create a brand with an excellent reputation. Normally, the branding process aims to be completely ethical, showing the consumer that because a company makes an excellent product, other products of the same brand can be expected to show the same high quality. However, arguably branding can take on a deceptive quality in which the properties of one product are expected to exert a halo effect on other products that are very different. Fast food companies tout their "healthy" options, partly to keep customers who have had to become more diet-conscious, but also to create a "healthy" image of the whole brand. The restaurant chain may still make the greatest amount of revenue on customers buying their core products such as high-fat burgers, but count on their healthy options to make their unhealthy meals seem not quite as gluttonous. Automobile companies have spent huge amounts of money on developing environmentally conscious electric vehicles that account for tiny fractions of their sales. Although the electric vehicle product lines consistently lose money, they are thought to exert a halo effect on the whole company's image, helping the company to gain customers for its core product lines. It is perhaps a stretch to believe that the properties of the electric car have any relevance to the decision to buy a large truck made by the same company. However, companies continue to believe, probably with good reason, that their electric cars are influencing the brand image and enhancing sales of their core product lines.

Applications in Medicine

The halo effect has many applications to patient satisfaction. Patients are usually poor at judging the physician's clinical skills, but easily form judgments of nonclinical aspects of the office visit, especially appearance and providers' interpersonal skills.[47] Imagine one office with a clean, tidy waiting room with complimentary coffee and a TV that is not too loud, a variety of magazines, courteous staff at the front desk, kind nurses with acceptable waiting time, and a physician wearing an ironed white coat, dress shirt, and acceptable dark colored socks. Now imagine a different office with rude staff, a dirty waiting room, and a slovenly, poorly dressed physician. Although the care provided by the physician in the second office may be highly competent and effective, the patient is likely to extrapolate from the appearance and decide that the care they received was substandard.[48] Meanwhile, in the attractive office, the patient may be prepared to overlook negative aspects of the visit because the appearance gives a clear impression of high quality and caring about the patient's needs (Table 1). Dan Ariely writes, "Every time we can't evaluate the real thing we are interested in, we find something easy to evaluate and make an inference based on it. I often hear people complain, for example, about the cleanliness of airplane bathrooms. The reality is that we don't really care about the bathrooms — what we should all care about is the functioning of the engines. But engines are hard to evaluate, so we focus on the bathrooms. Maybe people reason that if the airline is taking care of the bathrooms, it is probably taking care of the engines."[49] Since most patients do not have the knowledge to evaluate the physician's clinical skill accurately, physicians need to pay attention to the aspects that patients are more likely to actually judge them on, such as cleanliness.

Table 1. Office Evaluation Checklist[48] (Reproduced with permission of *The Dermatologist*.)

Waiting Room
___ Magazines are in good condition.
___ Water cooler cup dispenser is clean.
___ The trashcan is not next to the water cooler.
___ Roof panels are unstained.
___ The check-in desk is in good condition.
___ Patient flyers are on a bulletin board, not taped to windows.

__ All windowsills are clean.

Clinic Hallways

__ Entrance door is well maintained.

__ Nurses' Desk is well maintained.

__ Nurses' area is clean.

__ Patient folders are in good condition.

__ Wallpaper is well maintained.

__ No papers are taped to walls or doors.

__ All signs are laminated.

__ Exam room doors are clean.

__ Cryoablation device is not easily accessible to patients.

__ Patient folder holders are clean.

__ Dry-erase boards outside patient rooms are clean.

__ Pictures and frames are in good condition.

__ Hallways are generally clean and free of dust.

__ There are no scuff marks on the floors.

Exam Room

__ Wallpaper is well maintained.

__ There are no holes in the walls.

__ There is no writing on the walls.

__ There is no tape left on the walls.

__ No nails are showing in the wall.

__ Plastic information and folder holders are clean.

__ Sinks are clean.

__ Mirrors are clean.

__ Patient chair and footstool are clean.

__ Equipment tray is clean or covered with a clean drape.

__ Trash cans are well maintained.

__ Patient/visitor chairs are well maintained.

__ Coat hangers are well maintained.

__ Door knobs are clean.

__ All cabinets are well maintained.
__ All windowsills are clean.
__ Floors are clean.

Another application is that the importance of attractiveness in the way people are viewed may make "cosmetic" treatments more valuable than policymakers generally realize. Although acne and rosacea may not cause physical pain, patients feel that they are judged more negatively because of their acne or rosacea, which can be devastating. Due to prevailing myths that acne is caused by poor hygiene or that facial redness always indicates alcohol abuse, patients sense that they are assumed to be unhygienic or alcoholics, and suffer discrimination at work, school, or in dating. The halo effect of attractiveness may explain why the willingness to pay for acne and rosacea treatment is as high as for life-threatening conditions like hypertension.[50] The high value of attractiveness may explain why botulinum toxin procedures surprised observers by continuing to flourish even during the economic downturn following the 2008 financial crisis.[51]

Quick Tips

- Brands with excellent reputations exert halo effects, improving perception of all products bearing the same brand.
- Easily perceived attributes like the appearance of a medical office, or doctor's bedside manner, exert a halo effect on the overall visit.
- Aesthetic treatments can greatly improve quality of life due to the halo effect.

Chapter 10
Curse of Knowledge
Asmaa Al-Kadhi, Scott A. Davis, and Steven R. Feldman

The **Curse of Knowledge** is a cognitive bias where better-informed people find it extremely difficult to think from the perspective of lesser-informed people. The difficulty an expert faces in explaining a complex idea to a child or an uninformed person is an example.

The Curse of Knowledge affects our daily lives in many aspects: in the business world, in medicine and in teaching. Once we know something, we find it hard to imagine that others do not know it. Our knowledge has "cursed" us and we have difficulty explaining or teaching concepts to others who do not share the same experience and information background. If any of the material in this book has seemed opaque, that is likely a result of the Curse of Knowledge effect on the authors of that material.

Background and History
Although the idea behind the "Curse of Knowledge" appears to be self-evident, coining the term "Curse of Knowledge" is credited to Professor Robin M. Hogarth of the University of Chicago.[52]

Examples and Analysis
In 1990, Elizabeth Newton from Stanford University conducted an experiment in which a group of participants, called "tappers", were asked to finger tap on a table a melody

chosen from a list of twenty-five popular songs and melodies, like "Happy Birthday to You" and "The Star Spangled Banner" and another group, called "tappers", were asked to identify the songs being tapped.[53]

Before the experiment began, the tappers were asked how often they believed the listeners would correctly identify the tapped melodies. The tappers expected the listeners to identify one of every two (50%). In reality, the listeners identified only three out of the 120 songs tapped for them (2.5%).

The song was so clear in the tappers' minds; how could the listeners not "hear" it? When a tapper taps, he is hearing the song in his head. You can try it for yourself, tap out "Happy Birthday to You." It's impossible to avoid hearing the tune in your head. Meanwhile, the listeners cannot hear that tune; all they can hear is a bunch of disconnected taps, like a kind of incoherent Morse code. In the experiment, tappers were astonished at how hard the listeners seem to be working to pick up the tune.

The tappers have pre-existing information of the melody they tap that makes it difficult for them to imagine what it's like for the listeners, who hear isolated taps rather than a song. This is the Curse of Knowledge. Once we know something, we find it hard to imagine what it is like not to know it.

The Heath brothers, in their book *Made to Stick*, suggested that the more you know about a subject, the harder it often becomes to communicate your knowledge to someone who knows nothing about the topic.[54]

The Heath brothers' SUCCESs model seeks to overcome the Curse of Knowledge by thinking about your messages from an audience's perspective and how to make the ideas "sticky" for them.[55]

S: Simple: no need to use words difficult to understand, be clear and simple.

U: Unexpected: try to say something curious and out of line, surprise the listeners.

C: Concrete: try to link it to something memorable, by that it will stick in the listener's mind.

C: Credible: gain the trust of your listeners.

E: Emotional: involve your listener's emotions.

S: Stories: use stories to help people understand, stories will stick more than statistics.

Applications in Medicine

Medical doctors, specialized professionals, and any group of people (like certain hobbyists, video gamers...) who use a special set of terminology, not shared by the community at large, tend to be at a higher risk of falling victim to the Curse of Knowledge (Table 1). They usually forget that other people do not share their knowledge, experience or background.

In a series of medical encounters, physicians often did not tell the patient what the diagnosis was, what the treatment was supposed to do, how often to take the treatment, how much to use, and when to stop. Presumably the physicians knew all these issues so well that they didn't think to communicate them to their patients.

Even when doctors do explain these fundamental aspects of disease and its treatment, many people have difficulties understanding what their doctors are saying when the doctor builds his explanation on his own knowledge and experience, instead of doing so from the point of view of the patient. Awareness is the first step in dealing with any problem including the Curse of Knowledge. Acknowledging that the speaker and the audience may come from different backgrounds, and have a different area of knowledge and experience is very important.

It is good to remember that hearing a tune in your head does not make your audience hear the same tune automatically. In order for patients to learn from you about their condition, you will have to present your ideas in a way that your patients can understand. This way will often be very different from the way you and your colleagues think about the condition.

Table 1: Common misunderstandings and solutions for them

Possibly misunderstood action, statement, or word	Patient's interpretation	Better alternative
Diagnose psoriasis immediately upon walking in the room, because the diagnosis is obvious	Lesions were not closely examined; physician is uncaring[56]	Look at the lesions closely through a magnifying glass before stating the diagnosis

Not examine a potentially malignant lesion closely because you plan to biopsy it	Lesion was not closely examined; physician is uncaring	Look at the lesion through a magnifying glass, then biopsy
"Steroid"	Anabolic steroid ("what baseball players take to bulk up")	"Cortisone-type medication"
"Have you had a psychiatric condition?"	Craziness, insanity	"Have you had any depression or anxiety?"
"Have you had any GI problems?"	GI = soldier	"Have you had any problems with your stomach or digestion?"
"The test came back negative."	Negative means a bad result	"The test came back normal."
"You are going to see a resident."	May not understand that a resident is a more advanced trainee (not a student) and might demand to see only the faculty physician	Explain the resident is a physician and provide their qualifications

Quick Tips

- People who have specialized knowledge tend to forget what it is like not to have that knowledge.
- Never take for granted that your patients know how to use a treatment, how much to use, or when to stop.
- Be especially careful about using medical terms that have a different meaning to the lay public than they do for professionals.

PART II

Social Effects:
How Irrationality Affects the
Patient-Physician Relationship

Chapter 11
Submission and Resistance to Authority
Scott A. Davis and Steven R. Feldman

Every human society has authority figures. **Authority** is defined as the combination of power and legitimacy, the right to exercise the power. Humans seem programmed to favor extremes when choosing how to respond to authorities – either complete submission or determined resistance. Activating the automatic system of behavior for submitting to authority can sometimes be adaptive. (For more about automatic vs. reflective systems of behavior, see Chapter 1 of *Nudge*.[30]) For example, people who automatically submit when confronted by a police officer usually come out better off. However, in other situations, a middle-of-the-road, negotiated outcome is better, and the tendency toward the extremes of total submission or total resistance can be a drawback. In this chapter, we will examine human behavior toward authority figures, including physicians, and some undesired consequences of total submission or total resistance.

Background and History
The concept of authority is as old as human civilization. Although modern people may tend to react negatively to the idea of authority, the importance of strong authorities in society has been advocated by writers as eminent as Plato, Niccolo Machiavelli, Thomas Hobbes, and Friedrich Nietzsche. These thinkers emphasized benefits of strong authority such as wise rule by "philosopher-kings", political stability and unity, an end to the "war of all against all", and

sustaining the values of the superman. However, with the horrific record of war and genocide of 20th-century authoritarian regimes, the human tendency to follow authority has increasingly been questioned, and psychologists have tried to discover why people submit so readily to authorities even when tremendous evil results.

In the period following World War II, psychologists sought to answer the question of how so many people could have participated in the evils of the Nazi regime and Holocaust. They found that the tendency to follow authority was extremely widespread, even in ordinary people in democracies. Stanley Milgram showed that 65% of subjects would obey an experimenter by continuing to increase the level of what they believed to be an electric shock to the maximum, even once the victim cried out in intense pain.[57] Around the same time, Solomon Asch demonstrated that a participant in his study could be convinced to ignore their senses and assert that a line that was clearly longer than others was actually the shortest, provided that the whole group agreed that it was the shortest.[58] Asch noted that this conforming behavior was substantially reduced when just one other person agreed with the participant on the dissenting opinion. This finding may give support to a more hopeful view, in which a few brave individuals can speak up against a corrupt authority and show that the official opinion is not unanimous, leading others to switch sides. The fall of Soviet and East European communism may have been an example of this "house of cards" effect. A modest number of brave dissidents like Alexander Solzhenitsyn and Vaclav Havel, with the support of a few widely respected figures like Pope

John Paul II of Poland, were able to show that the support for communist parties was very shallow and could collapse quickly.

Examples and Analysis

The neuropsychology of individuals' relationship to authority is not surprising given the human tendency to be a cognitive miser (i.e. to avoid expending more than a minimum of mental effort and instead use mental shortcuts). Noreena Hertz writes that the brain can shut off completely when faced with an expert sharing expert knowledge.[59] Rather than integrating the new information with old information, the brain often seems to make a binary decision to accept the expert's knowledge completely, or ignore it. If the expert is perceived as a hostile authority figure, the brain will tend to shift into a mode of total resistance. Hertz notes that this effect is especially strong when the expert is giving bad news that the listener would rather ignore (see Chapter 20, Ostrich effect).[59] Hence, Hertz writes, "If [smokers'] unconscious belief is that they won't get lung cancer, for every warning from an antismoking campaigner, their brain is giving a lot more weight to that story of the 99-year-old lady who smokes 50 cigarettes a day but is still going strong."[59]

In this case, the antismoking campaigner is also likely to be perceived as a member of an outgroup who does not understand the feelings and preferences of smokers. Much political discourse draws its effectiveness from labeling an opponent as a member of a hostile outgroup with evil motives.[60] Often the biggest gaffe a politician can make in American politics is coming across as "out of touch" with the average voter, invoking the voter's hostile outgroup response. People with strong partisan identification are likely not even listening to the arguments of a politician from another party, but their brains have already shifted into a mode of automatically rejecting whatever they hear.

However, the person who provokes a resistant response is not always from an outgroup, but can even be a family member that we love. As soon as one family member asks another to take out the trash, the second person's instinctive response is often, "No, you can't <u>make</u> me do it!" In psychology, this behavior is called reactance, and is especially evident when a strongly worded message seems to constrain a person's freedom greatly.[61, 62] Therefore, reactance theorists recommend that health-promoting messages should avoid controlling language and end with a statement reassuring the recipient that they remain free to choose.[62] Miller et al. found that a short postscript appearing to restore the listener's freedom to choose can be surprisingly effective, even if the rest of the message is quite different.[62]

On the other hand, if an expert is trusted, total submission is often the brain's automatic response. Automatic submission to the government or one's boss may sometimes be a logical response, but at the other extreme, it can lead to bad behavior that people excuse on the grounds of "just following orders". This excuse is known as the Nuremberg defense, after its use by Nazi officials who defended themselves in the Nuremberg Trials by saying they were just following the orders of Hitler. Although international law has now made it clear that the Nuremberg defense is not a legitimate defense in cases of war crimes, many people still obey unethical orders for fear of retribution. A recent example was the massive cover-up in the Penn State sex abuse scandal, where several witnesses who could have spoken up much earlier remained silent. The prestige enjoyed by the Penn State football program was so great that people feared being ostracized by the entire town if they exposed criminal behavior by the leaders of this once-revered institution.

Applications in Medicine
Although not resulting in such profoundly harmful and immoral behavior as in other contexts, automatic submission to medical experts can preclude optimal exchange of information between patient and physician. Patients adopting a posture of total submission might not be so bad if we had 100% of the relevant information about the patient's situation and preferences, but this is almost never the case (Table 1). Neither party actually has a monopoly on relevant knowledge; patients are the expert on their personal experience of illness and their own preferences and values, while we bring greater medical and therapeutic knowledge.[63] Nonetheless, patients may view the relationship as lopsided with all the expertise on our side, and often feel it is very natural to be totally submissive. We therefore have a responsibility to ensure that the patient does not lapse into the total submission mode.

Relationship	Risk factors	Impact on treatment plan	Consequences
Total submission	Depressive disorder	*Physician's input: 100%* *Patient's input: 0%* Patient's perspective is left unstated and physician cannot take it into account.	*Passive resistance*: Patient is prescribed a treatment that is out of line with their preferences. May feel a polite "white lie" to the doctor – saying that they are following the treatment plan – is the socially acceptable thing to do. May feel it would take chutzpah to "talk back" to a person with very high IQ and white coat!
Total resistance	Antisocial personality disorder, adolescence [56]	*Physician's input: 0%* *Patient's input: 100%* Patient ignores advice, having already made a decision that the physician's recommendations are unacceptable.	*Reactance*: Patient becomes determined to defy the physician and resist perceived restrictions on their freedom, thus does not follow the treatment plan

Respectful negotiation		*Both parties have significant input* Patient and physician can settle on a mutually agreeable treatment plan.	Patient believes the treatment plan was "their idea" and is motivated to follow it. Trust and sense of a common goal are enhanced.

Table 1. Potential results of overly submissive, overly resistant, or optimal behavior. Although total submission and total resistance may seem like complete opposites, their consequences may be much the same. The patient cannot unilaterally impose a treatment plan that is unacceptable to the physician, but holds effective veto power over the physician's plan with the threat of nonadherence.

A respectful give-and-take can begin with eliciting features that the patient believes are important in a treatment.[64] The patient can be asked to state on a scale of 1 to 10 how motivated they are to achieve certain health goals, leading the patient to state factors that enhance or limit their motivation to work toward the goal.[65] For example, a patient may say, "Well, I don't like to use sunscreen because it is messy when I'm doing sweaty work, and I'm able to get my actinic keratoses frozen off every year at your office, so what is the point?" This statement may reveal that sun-protective clothing is a more realistic option for this patient.

Whether the patient's initial posture is total submission, total resistance, or somewhere in between, causing the patient to feel that the plan was their own idea is very helpful. We can offer several options, and the patient can choose one that feels like a personal choice. If the patient hesitates when presented with multiple options, it may become apparent that the patient is not comfortable with any of the options and wants to suggest something completely different.

For patients prone to total resistance, we will need to make an extra effort to establish a sense of connection and common interest. A question such as, "What do you like about smoking?" asked sincerely and nonjudgmentally, may jolt the patient out of total resistance mode. Once the patient has given an honest answer, it may be possible to brainstorm healthier ways to get similar benefits. If a patient is determined not to take a specific medication, we may be able to offer comforting words upon hearing the patient's horror story about the medication. The patient may be pleasantly surprised that a physician finally took the time to listen to their story. The patient may also be impressed that we understood the hidden meaning behind the question; for example, "Is this a steroid?" in an anxious tone of voice really means, "Is this safe for my child?" Building on this trust, we can recommend an alternative option, emphasizing its differences from the disliked medication. If a patient is determined not to take medication at all, there may be other treatments or lifestyle interventions that accommodate this preference. According to reactance theory, adding a concluding message showing that we support the patient's freedom of choice, especially if we sense that we have been lecturing them too much, may be helpful.

Quick Tips

- Humans tend to choose either automatic submission or automatic resistance to authority figures.
- Very submissive patients need to be empowered to express their perspective so that we may take it into account.
- Resistant patients benefit when we make a connection and consider their objections fairly, such as listening to an experience that gave them a negative view of a treatment.

Chapter 12
Resisting ideas of others
Imran Aslam, Scott A. Davis, and Steven R. Feldman

Newton's first law of motion essentially states that objects are resistant to change unless acted upon by an outside force. Humans, like objects, are also resistant to change, except that humans are more likely to change if they are "acted upon" by an internal force as opposed to an external one. The idea and motivation to change must come from within, for people have a strong tendency to favor and support their own ideas, while also exhibiting a **tendency to resist the ideas of others**.[66] This latter aspect is especially true when external ideas imposed on an individual pose a threat to autonomy. The reflexive tendency to resist external demands and preserve autonomy is deeply instilled in human nature and presents a problem because it may reduce patients' participation in recommended treatment. This tendency can, on the other hand, be harnessed to promote patients' wellbeing. In chapter 11 we introduced the topic of resistance, and in this chapter we will continue our discussion in greater detail while exploring potential solutions.

Background and History
Our body's immune system has a remarkable defense mechanism that functions by impulsively attacking foreign invaders. This defense mechanism helps to prevent many diseases and infections; yet in certain instances, such as transplant procedures, it can be counterproductive. That is why it is possible to avoid detection by the immune system by

coating foreign particles with self protein, and thus avoiding imminent attack. This phenomenon is analogous to our cognitive defense system that functions similarly by resisting foreign ideas. And just like the immune system, this cognitive defense system can be bypassed by framing ideas in a manner such that the individual can adopt it is as his own. This very principle constitutes the foundation for motivational interviewing. Motivational interviewing (MI) is not a means of deceiving people into doing something that they don't want to do; "rather it is a skillful clinical style for eliciting from patients their own good motivations for making behavior changes in the interest of their health."[67] MI is a counseling technique that originated in 1983 and was initially developed to help overcome alcohol addiction. This technique uses a style of interviewing that is supportive and goal directed in order to elicit behavior modification. The patient is guided by the clinician to identify problematic behavior and then the patient is encouraged to express potential changes he can make.[68]

MI uses a series of questions to help patients progress their thinking. Patients may start at a point where they are not considering change and then through the use of directed question they can be led to a point where they are ready to consider change. In order to further illustrate this here is an example of a series of questions that works up to a specific goal.

Do you think readers already know what MI is?
Do you think that it is important for readers to understand what MI is?
Do you think they would understand it better if you gave them an example of it?

Do you think it might be good to add somewhere among these paragraphs an example table or figure that showed a series of questions that would illustrate for them what MI is and how it would be used?

Another example of MI in the school setting could potentially be a counselor-student meeting aimed at helping the student improve his grades by addressing his tendency to procrastinate. According to MI, the counselor's first task would be to help the student acknowledge that there is a problem. The counselor could start this discussion by asking the student "what brings you in to see me today?" Once the student demonstrates understanding of his predicament, the counselor can move on to assess the student's willingness to change by stating "I understand you are having some difficulty in school, is this an area of concern for you?" If the student is concerned and interested in changing, then the next step would be for the counselor to guide the student to identify the troublesome behavior of procrastination and articulate a plan of action. MI requires the counselor to move at the pace of the student, to resist the urge to instruct, and to allow the student to do the heavy lifting of verbalizing the problem and proposing the solution.

MI has also demonstrated its value in a variety of clinical scenarios that require behavior modification. It is effective at improving patient adherence to glucose monitoring, improving medication usage, and decreasing alcohol and illicit drug use.[67] For this reason studies using MI in the management of hypertension, cardiovascular disease, diabetes, and pathologic gambling have also reported encouraging outcomes.[67] One of the reasons MI is successful is because it accounts for the human tendency to resist the ideas of others. William Miller, the founder of MI, acknowledges in his book that in order to elicit behavior change one must understand that "there is something in human nature that resists being coerced and told what to do. Ironically it is acknowledging the other's right not to change that sometimes makes change possible."[67] This principle also relates back to the concept of reactance which was discussed in chapter 11.

When discussing MI it is important to consider intrinsic versus extrinsic motivation. Intrinsic motivation is any activity that is done for its innate satisfaction, while extrinsic motivation is an activity done for some external reward. [69] In MI the goal is to help individuals realize all potential motivations for behavior change, whether it is intrinsic, extrinsic or both. The advantage of intrinsic motivation is that it produces a long lasting effect, and by definition does not require a system of punishments or rewards. Extrinsic motivation, on the other hand, tends to be short lived and requires incentives. From a MI standpoint it is easier to facilitate the identification of extrinsic motivations; whereas, fostering intrinsic motivation tends to be a more tedious process.[70]

Another phenomenon that coincides with our discussion of resisting ideas of others is the generation effect. The generation effect is the phenomenon where information tends to be more memorable when it is generated by an individual rather than when it is provided by an outside source.[71] One of the early experiments demonstrated this by showing increased retention in subjects who had to generate the word rabbit from a word fragment (e.g., "r-bb-t") compared to subjects who just read the actual word.[72] Deriving information in areas such as mathematics, reading comprehension, and trivia are more memorable than just passive reading or listening.[71] A practical application of the generation effect observed during exam preparation would be to rephrase important concepts.[73] This technique forces an individual to become an active learner and makes the material more memorable than if it were just read. Another application of the generation effect in the classroom setting would be to have questions integrated into book chapters. This addition would encourage students to refer back to the previously read text and would reinforce important concepts while contributing to an overall more interactive experience.

Examples and Analysis

The tendency to resist the ideas of others is a common pattern in human behavior that can be observed throughout history. The understanding of this tendency can be used to further contextualize many major historical events including the American Revolution. One of the major reasons the American Revolution occurred can be summarized by the slogan "No taxation without representation." The problem the British colonists had with King George III was not that he was taxing them, but that he was taxing them without representing them. Had the king asked the colonists how they wanted to pay for the expense of governing them, perhaps there would have been no war. Many wars start this way. Country A makes an ultimatum, which shifts the frame of the argument within Country B to, "Who do they think they are, telling us what to do?!" Once this point is reached, a peaceful solution becomes unlikely. The essence of many conflicts whether on a national level or an individual one can be traced back to this type of resistance.

Families with adolescent aged individuals are all too familiar with the episodes of conflict that stem from a source of underlying teenage resistance. Many parents grow frustrated with their adolescent children when they blatantly break rules and test boundaries. Adolescents may come home after curfew, skip homework assignments, or get foolish piercings and body art that leave parents scratching their head wondering as to what went wrong. Part of the reason adolescents break rules is because rules are imposed on them, and in order to win back some of their autonomy they resist these ideas and act out. A potential strategy to improve adherence and reduce conflict would entail parent and child collaboration when deciding upon rules. For instance, parents could initiate a discussion by asking kids what they think a reasonable curfew would be, and then proceed to negotiate a reasonable time that hopefully satisfies both parties. The utility of this strategy lies in accounting for the tendency to resist by returning some control and autonomy back to children. It also enables a smoother transition to adulthood once the child turns 18 and is no longer bound by the parent's authority.

Granting children a sense of autonomy and control can go a long way at improving the relationships within a household. This principle can also be applied beyond the home to improve the workplace as well. According to the job characteristics model, autonomy was found to be one of the five qualities that can improve employee motivation, satisfaction, and performance.[74, 75] This model demonstrates the role autonomy plays in motivating individuals. When an adolescent is given the autonomy to set his own curfew he is more motivated to actually follow it. The same holds true in the corporate world; employees that are granted autonomy in decision- making will feel an overall greater sense of responsibility and motivation. A U.S. printing company tried this strategy of increasing worker autonomy by creating independent teams and found that employees worked harder, utilized a greater skill set, and demonstrated a greater aptitude for problem solving.[76]

Applications in Medicine

Motivating employees or helping an individual find the motivation to change is not an easy task. Many people have certain behaviors or habits that they know are bad for them and wish to change; yet, they struggle to find the motivation to do so. Behaviors such as smoking, excessive alcohol use, and poor diet are hard to break, but may benefit from MI. MI is based on "four guiding principles: 1) resist the righting reflex 2) understand and explore the person's own motivations 3) listen with empathy 4) to empower the individual, encouraging hope and optimism."[67] These principles serve as a lesson for clinicians and non-clinicians alike on how to interact with anyone trying to change. For instance, according to these principles, smokers should not be chastised, but instead they should be encouraged to articulate their feelings about quitting and the challenges they face. By offering an empathetic ear and words of support and hope we can help any individual find the motivation to change.

These principles of MI are invaluable when applied to one on one situations; however, they aren't as practical when addressing larger groups of people. A different approach to behavior change can be seen marketed to mass audiences via promotional health messages. Promotional health messages encouraging exercise, dieting, pro breastfeeding, and anti-smoking seem to be on the rise over television, radio, and other media outlets in recent years. It is an optimistic sign to see that there is finally an alternative voice competing with the overwhelming pro fast food, candy, and alcohol related messages that plague our media today. With that said, it is critical that we use our voice in healthcare tactfully in order to get the most bang for our buck. Tact is especially important when considering promotional health messages directed at the adolescent population. This population can be highly resistant and rebellious to overtly strong messages that "tell them what to do." Previous research indicates that "intense, forceful, or dogmatic language may increase the magnitude of reactance."[61] Furthermore, a study by Grandpre et al. demonstrated that high school students exposed to forceful antismoking messages were more likely to resist and attempt smoking. Additionally, the reverse was also true: when students were exposed to a strong, overly persuasive pro-smoking message, they were more likely to reject smoking.[62, 77] I am not advising that we start pro-smoking campaigns in schools across the nation; however, it may help to recognize resistance and carefully phrase health messages to avoid sounding overtly explicit or forceful especially when targeting highly resistant populations.

Another challenge with the adolescent population from the healthcare perspective is medication compliance.[78] A previous study examined strategies to improve compliance in adolescents with acne vulgaris. This study found that the group of adolescents whose parents received daily phone calls telling them, "Don't forget! Remind your child to use the medication," had significantly worse compliance rates than the group that received no daily reminders.[79] Another related study found the use of daily text message reminders to be ineffective at improving adherence to topical acne medication.[80] It can be theorized that the daily reminders may have been perceived as irritating and triggered a sense of resistance in the adolescent subjects, thereby reducing compliance.[79] On the other hand, a weekly Internet survey, which made patients feel that the doctor anticipated obstacles they were already thinking about, nearly tripled adherence to the medication.[81] These studies further reinforce the importance of being cognizant of the resistance phenomenon when treating our patients and delivering promotional health messages.

One of the approaches that we could employ to avoid resistance in our patients would be to frame treatment options in such a way that the patient adopts it as his or her own idea. For instance this discussion could start with the open ended question, "What is important to you in a treatment?" If the patient has difficulty with generating a response, progress to a more directed question allowing the patient to choose among options, such as, "Do you prefer a treatment that gets rid of your symptoms as fast as possible, or one that works slower but has fewer side effects?" By facilitating and engaging patients in this dialogue we can foster a sense of responsibility and motivation to adhere to treatment regimens. This becomes possible when the treatment decision is no longer "our" idea but theirs.

Once patients take ownership of their treatment plan they are more likely to abide by it; however, there will still be times when patients simply forget to take their medications. This is a common obstacle faced in healthcare today, and is quite understandable especially when complex medical regimens are superimposed on already hectic lives. Therefore, it would be beneficial to help patients develop a strategy to remember their medications. Of course, for reasons we have already discussed, it is important that these strategies be elicited from the patient, not imposed on them by us. For example, instead of telling patients to take their medicine at the same time each day, to ask them "what time of day did you decide to take the medication at?" Another possible strategy could be to ask patients "which of the following methods would you prefer as a way to remember to take your medication? A. Pill box B. Electronic reminder C. Post it note D. Family member or E. other." To the extent that we can, it may be worthwhile to implement practical strategies such as these examples to help improve patient compliance.

Once we are ready to conclude our patient visit it is a good idea to ensure patient understanding by employing the teach back method. This technique requires patients to express what they have understood and what they plan to do and will further invite any potential questions that need to be addressed.[82] This technique functions similar to how students remember more when they are required to teach others about a topic they just learned. The teach back method as well as the other techniques mentioned in this section will help us better anticipate and avoid resistance to hopefully improve compliance and better serve our patients.

Assess willingness to change[83]

Clinician: How important would you say changing your drinking is right now?

Client: Not very.

Clinician: Why do you say that?

Client: I have so many other worries about my health.

Clinician: It seems to you that your drinking is not the most important thing right now. What would have to happen to make it more important?

Client: I think if I had another DUI and lost my driver's license that might get my attention

Plan of Action

Clinician: What do you think you'll do about changing your drinking? What ideas do you have for yourself?

Client: I'm not sure. I could try what my best friend is doing, to go to one AA meeting just to see what it's like.

Sample MI questions for clinician use:[84]

	Sample questions
Identifying problem	How does your (lack of a GED/using drugs/alcohol/peers) fit in with your goals? On one hand you say your (Health/Children) are important to you, however, you continue to (Drink/Use Drugs/get arrested) , help me to understand…. How is being unemployed working for you? And/or your family? How will things be for you a year from now if you continue to _____? But, how is this a problem for YOU? Do you agree with what they say? Do you think that these things will ever happen to you?
Provide support	You've done well to have survived all of that… I can tell this has really bothered you…
Life Goals	What sorts of things are important to you? What do you see yourself doing in a year

	from now? Once off probation, what do you see as the ideal situation for you? What is it going to take for you to have the ideal situation?
Plan of action	You were saying that you were trying to decide whether you should continue or cut down… Tell me about your decision? What is it you would like to do?

Quick Tips

- Motivational interviewing provides tools to help patients develop a plan that they feel is their own idea.
- Reactance suggests that people react strongly to protect their freedom of choice when confronted with a behavior change message.
- To improve adherence, ask, "How would <u>you</u> go about remembering to take the medication regularly?"

PART III

Emotional Effects:
How Emotions Influence Our View
of Health and Treatments

Chapter 13

Loss Aversion

Scott A. Davis, Asmaa Al-Kadhi, and Steven R. Feldman

Loss aversion is the tendency to place a greater value on losses than gains of comparable size. In research studies, to get average subjects to accept even odds on a bet with a possible $5 loss, a $10 potential gain needs to be offered. And while people dislike taking risks (people are more likely to accept a sure gain over a gamble offering a potential greater gain), people may still take risks to avoid losses (figure 1). Loss aversion is different from risk aversion, since a person who is risk averse would be expected to choose a guaranteed smaller loss (choice D in Figure 1) instead of taking a risk to avoid a larger loss (choice C).

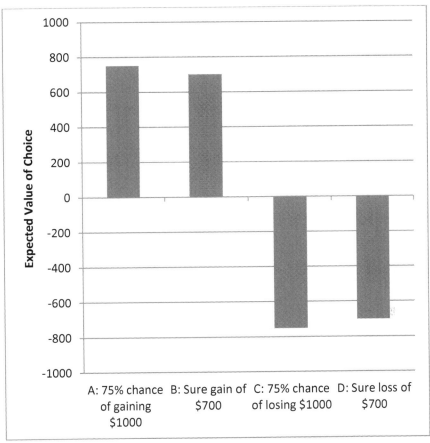

Figure 1. Although both violate strict rational-choice theory, loss aversion is different from risk aversion. Under both loss aversion and risk aversion, B is preferred over A. However, the majority of people show a preference for the loss-averse choice C over the risk-averse choice D, since C offers a chance to avoid losing anything.

Background and History
Loss aversion was described by Daniel Kahneman and Amos Tversky in 1984.[1] In one experiment, 72% of study subjects preferred a disease-prevention program that would definitely

save 200 lives over one that had a 1/3 chance of saving 600 lives. When the choice was presented in terms of lives lost, only 22% preferred a program that caused 400 lives to be lost over one that had a 1/3 chance of no lives lost.[1] The two sets of choices are mathematically identical (Figure 2), but emphasizing lives lost greatly increased the degree of risk-seeking. Similar experiments showed that as in Figure 1, people were willing to accept a risky choice to avoid a loss, even when the expected value of the risky choice was a greater loss. However, when a gain was offered, people avoided risky choices and accepted a sure gain even when the expected value of a risky option was greater. The results showed that two fundamental assumptions of rational choice theorists – that preferences should not be influenced by the presentation of a question, and that a choice with a higher expected value should always be preferred – did not hold in many circumstances.

Framing 1
Do you prefer

Framing 2
Do you prefer

Option 1A:
100% chance
of saving 200
lives

Option 2A:
100% chance
of losing 400
lives

OR

OR

Option 1B:
1/3 chance of
saving 600
lives

Option 2B:
1/3 chance of
losing no lives

AND

AND

2/3 chance of
saving no
lives?

2/3 chance of
losing 600
lives?

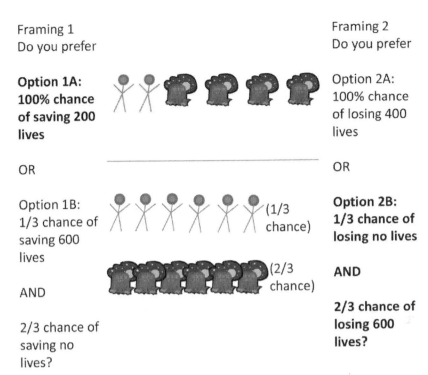

(1/3 chance)

(2/3 chance)

Figure 2. In Framing 1, the majority of subjects preferred Option 1A since the baseline for comparison was no lives saved, making 1A appear as a "safe" gain. In Framing 2, the majority preferred Option 2B since the baseline was no lives lost, making the risky option desirable to have a chance to avoid the loss. In fact, as the graphic shows, Options 1A and 2A are mathematically identical, and Options 1B and 2B are also mathematically identical.

Examples and Analysis

Framing has a powerful impact on whether people view events as gains, losses, or another category, such as costs. Increasing one's retirement savings contribution when receiving a pay raise is less painful than increasing it at another time, when it would result in a decrease in take-home pay.[30] For example, if workers receive a 5% raise, they can change their retirement savings contribution from 0 to 5% and keep the same take-home paycheck. If they wanted to raise their retirement savings contribution at another time, they would experience a 5% drop in take-home pay, which would probably require reducing their budget for everyday expenditures and cause loss aversion. The Save More Tomorrow program takes advantage of this concept by asking workers to agree in advance that they will increase their contributions when they get raises.[30]

The theory of loss aversion also states that people are more likely to accept negative events that are framed as a cost rather than a loss.[1] In an experiment by Slovic, Fischhoff, and Lichtenstein, 80% of subjects preferred a 25% chance of losing $200 over a sure loss of $50, but only 35% preferred not to pay the $50 when it was framed as insurance against the 25% chance of losing $200.[85] This simple reframing dramatically alters preferences. Another example is that in the past, individual investors rarely bought stock options, but when they started to view put options (which rise when the market falls) as insurance against market downturns, the popularity of these options soared. Options ceased to be simply a risky vehicle for speculators and day traders to seek outsized gains, and became a way to increase safety.

The idea of the dead-loss effect says that people are especially eager to avoid total loss of an investment, so they may go to great lengths to persuade themselves that an amount spent was a cost rather than a loss. A classic example was a man who continued to play tennis long after developing great pain from tennis elbow, rather than forfeit the membership fee he had already paid to belong to the tennis club.[40] By continuing to play tennis, he maintained his view of the membership fee as a cost, whereas if he had stopped playing, he would have been forced to view it as a loss.

More recently, Novemsky and Kahneman have refined the theory to suggest that loss aversion does not occur when a good is given up as intended, such as by a seller who intends to make money from selling the good, or when an item is being replaced by a newer and better version (Table 1).[86] Loss aversion is likely to be more profound for consumers who have strict budgets, who then have to take money out of a different account to cover the loss (see Chapter 7, Mental accounting). For very frugal consumers, Novemsky and Kahneman suggest reframing the purchase as an investment in a highly durable good that will last a long time, a view that helps justify reallocating money from the consumer's savings budget to buy the good.[86] This may be an important tactic in medicine since many patients do not anticipate needing healthcare expenditures, and do not budget for them in advance.

Table 1. Situations in which loss aversion is more or less likely to occur[86]

More likely
• Consumer must reallocate money from a different "mental account"
• Consumer has a strict budget with all income budgeted for a specific category of consumption or savings

Less likely
• The good is intended to be given up or sold for a profit
• A newly purchased good replaces the good being lost, without a time delay and sharing all the benefits of the lost good (e.g. an old car is traded in when buying a new one)
• Consumer has a flexible budget with available money not allocated for a specific purpose

Applications in Medicine

A drug will be viewed much more positively if it is said to prevent someone from dying a year earlier, rather than causing them to live a year longer. Framing the event as a loss of a year should thus be more impactful in getting the patient to use the drug.

Another implication of loss aversion is that patients may have a bias toward accepting less treatment than they would if they were not loss averse. Some patients are extremely reluctant to accept treatments with potential side effects, even if the side effect causes less suffering than the disease. It may be heartbreaking for a physician to see a patient who appears to be making the choice to continue suffering rather than try an effective treatment. When a patient manifests these preferences, we may want to frame the patient's choice in such a way that it is between two losses, rather than a loss and a gain. We may want to say, "This drug can prevent your disease from getting worse," rather than emphasizing the gain from remission of current symptoms. Faced with the expectation that their disease may get worse, patients may be prepared to take a risk to avoid the loss.

Dead-loss represents a sunk cost, that which has already been spent. Patients' aversion to dead-losses may be put to good use if the patient has already made considerable investment of time and money in seeking treatment or in activities that are jeopardized by the disease symptoms. If the patient has a gym membership they are not using, we might say, "It seems like it would be frustrating to waste your gym membership because of your psoriasis. If we clear up your condition with this medicine, you won't have to have wasted the gym membership fee." Similarly, for patients with insurance, we can emphasize that the patient has already paid for the insurance and should use the medication so they do not waste the valuable benefit they are entitled to.

Despite some recent improvement, undertreatment remains common in dermatology. The impetus for undertreatment can come from the physician, not just the patient. Fear of potential losses could preclude recommending treatments that have a high likelihood of providing benefit. We need to realize the consequences of our own cognitive biases that may lead us to recommend treatments that are not adequate to manage patients' conditions, leaving patients suffering.
Loss aversion can also be used to communicate the importance of healthy behaviors more forcefully. To increase patients' use of sunscreen and decrease use of tanning beds, the threat of losing the youthful beauty of patients' skin can be emphasized. Perhaps citing an example of a celebrity who lost her youthful appearance very quickly would be even more convincing. As we will see in Chapter 23, Hyperbolic Discounting, these approaches are more effective than emphasizing long term risks, such as skin cancer, that occurs decades later, as future events tend to be heavily discounted

in perceived importance.

Quick Tips

- People are often willing to make risky choices to avoid potential losses, which affect well-being more than gains.
- Emphasizing losses, such as loss of youthful beauty, may help persuade patients to follow healthier behaviors.
- Emphasizing a dead loss, such as money already invested in buying health insurance, may help overcome reluctance to take medication.

Chapter 14
Negativity Bias
Sandhya Chowdary, Scott A. Davis, and Steven R. Feldman

Negativity Bias is the propensity to attend to, learn from, and use negative information far more than positive information.[87]

Background & History:
"The evil that men do lives after them; the good is oft interred with their bones."- *Shakespeare*
Negative events influence our minds much more than positive events. Be it a negative trait, a bad day at work or a low-scoring report card, their after-effects tarnish one's self image for a long time to come. Often psychology scholars have pondered over this negative mindset that bad has a more powerful effect on perception than does good [88].

This tendency is consistent with Darwin's theory of 'survival of the fittest'. Both human and the animal species are more sensitive to bad experiences as it teaches them to avoid these in the future. Danger poses a threat to survival and the mind has to learn to 'expect' bad situations in order to protect the species, assuring longevity.

Memories of bad events take longer to wear off than good ones [89]. A study compared the effects of good and bad events on three groups of people. One group had won a lottery, one group had been paralyzed in an accident and the last group did not experience any major life event. The group that won the lottery were no happier than they were before winning it.

Time did not change the way they viewed life. The happiness of winning was not long lasting. On the other hand, the group that was paralyzed in an accident were unable to recover fully from the terrible aftermath of the incident until years later. They continued to compare their current life to life before the accident ("the nostalgia effect"). At 1 month to 1 year after the accident, they were less happy than the participants who had not experienced any major life changing event (the control group). Earlier, we noted in the discussion of the Tesla car fires that negative events are more salient than positive ones (See Chapter 4, Salience).

Negativity bias effects can be subclassified [90], including:

a. Negative Potency: A negative event has a more powerful effect on the human mind than a positive event. Humans tend to dwell more on negative influences than positive ones. For example, one scandal can overshadow a lifetime of public service as in the case of industrious, highly educated politicians like Eliot Spitzer and Richard Nixon.

b. Greater Steepness of Negative Gradients: Negative events grow more rapidly in negativity in space and time as compared to positive events. They tend to 'snowball' into a magnitude which affects human psychology in a harmful manner. Additional negative inputs have greater psychological effects than additional positive inputs. For instance, a series of bad relationships may adversely affect the mental status of a person even if they are presently in a stable and loving relationship. Somehow, the good from this current relationship cannot easily mitigate the harm done from the previous ones.

c. Negative dominance: When negative and positive events are added up together, the negative event takes predominance and is greater than the effect of each individual event.

It is the most important type of negativity bias and perhaps provides the greatest insight to the human thought process.

This is further divided into a *synchronic type* where the negative and positive events are occurring simultaneously and the negative event is disproportionately more influential. e.g. the good and bad traits of a person where the bad seems to overshadow the good. There is also a *diachronic type* where a positive event is cancelled out by a negative event. e.g. delicious food is perceived as inedible once an insect has come in contact with it whereas placing one's favorite food on top of a pile of insects hardly makes it edible.

On the same note, the term 'Contagion' was introduced. Literally meaning 'contamination', it implies that negative events leave behind their trace for a longer period of time and can penetrate into various sections of society indefinitely. For instance, in the Hindu culture, contact with a lower caste can contaminate a higher caste individual instantaneously whereas there is no limit to the number of rituals needed to completely purify a person.

d. <u>Greater Negative Differentiation</u>: Negative stimuli are more elaborately described and given more salience than positive stimuli. e.g. the vocabulary for negative emotions sound more prolific and emphatic as compared with positive emotions, the face has more expressions for displeasure than for pleasure or happiness.

Unfavorable information deters sales of a product [91].Favorable information is insufficient to offset any negative effect the unfavorable information had.

Physiological basis of Negativity Bias

The human mind has a heightened sensitivity to trouble and danger. Negative stimuli produce more neural activity, especially in the amygdala of the brain, than equally intense positive stimuli

Examples of Negativity Bias

a. A single item of negative information is capable of neutralizing five similar pieces of positive information [92]. A survey conducted on a group of psychology students revealed that an average of 25 lives would have to be saved in order to justify the murder of one person [90].

b. Negative publicity can severely damage a company's image where even after two weeks, people remember the negative statements written about it [93]. A study done on 91 people showed that negative press reports have long-lasting emotional and social consequences on the subjects reading them [94].

c. At the end of the day, we tend to think of the one thing

that went wrong rather than the numerous things that went right. As the adage goes, *"The brain is like Velcro for negative experiences, but Teflon for positive ones."* [95]

d. Political campaigns paint a negative picture of the opposing party rather than projecting a positive image of themselves. They make the general public fear that the worst will happen if they vote for the opposition e.g. higher taxes, higher insurance premiums.

e. It takes one act of violence or lack of discernment to ruin a marriage but many acts of forgiveness or kindness to rebuild it. Studies show that negative reciprocity among couples in the early stages of marriage have higher divorce rates later on. On the other hand, being loving and happy in the early stages does not guarantee a lower divorce rate in the later stages [88].

f. A child will need many words of encouragement to replace a single statement of discouragement or shame.

g. Consumers tend to pay more attention to negative reviews when purchasing a product. Though the quality of the product is excellent overall, the consumer's perception of it is tainted by scattered negative reviews [91].

Antidote to negativity bias

Studies have shown a few ways to at least partially circumvent negativity bias:

- Highly involved, loyal customers will mitigate the negative factors and take them less seriously than the regular customers [93].

- Corrective response and making necessary changes in a product increases its sales. Direct denial of the negative feedback received has an adverse effect on the sales of a product[96].

Though the cerebral cortex is sensitive to negative stimuli, our long-term memory has a tendency to retain positive information. Apparently, there are compensatory processes working to selectively recall positive memories e.g. recollecting fond memories of one's childhood despite the hardships of growing up [90].

Applications in Medicine

A patient may be more concerned about the side effects of the medication than the relief it will bring from the illness. The physician could explain the side effects with the help of visual aids/graphs showing that the side effects are minimal compared to the beneficial effects.

For example, biological therapies like etanercept are associated rarely with malignancy. Patients may focus on the rare association — even if it is not a causal relationship — and be terrified of the drug. Also, when the patient has heard a horror story about a medication from a friend, they will be reluctant to try it.

This negativity bias can also affect the perception of physicians who might inordinately fear a potentially beneficial therapy due to the rare side effects with which it may be associated.

Patients might recall a single discouraging statement or an inappropriate facial expression made by their physician. This may impact their feedback of the physician though his/her knowledge and bedside manner may be superior. Sometimes, physicians fail to realize that communication skills are often more important than the diagnosis itself. These "soft skills" are often overlooked in medical school in the exhausting race to complete a rigorous academic syllabus [97].

But patients are silent observers of our face and body language. Even paralinguistic speech characteristics such as speech rate, loudness, pitch and pauses in the physician's dialogue affect the patient. Non-verbal cues influence patients more often than verbal information. If the physician verbally reassures the patient saying, "You will be fine" but frowns while saying this, the patient is immediately concerned. A blank expression is equally unwelcoming to a patient as it communicates disinterest and lack of empathy on the part of the physician. Head nodding, eye contact, smiling and forward lean are few positive gestures that have gained positive feedback from patients.[98] Alcoholic patients refuse follow up treatment as they sensed hostility in the voice of their physician.[99]

To avoid negativity bias taking place in a patient's mind regarding the treatment plan, a good rapport should be established between the physician and patient. A "loyal" patient is far more open to the idea of trying a novel therapeutic agent because a relationship of trust has been built over time. This patient might even ignore negative reviews about the physician as there is enough positive to override it. Also if negative feedback is received from a patient, the physician should respond in a non-defensive manner. They may even go one step further and ask the patient to offer suggestions on how to improve their practice.

Quick Tips

*maybe ask my other patients who did decide to take it
to see if they're willing to share with those who are
reluctant*

- Patients are very reluctant to try some treatments because it takes many positive stories about a treatment to outweigh one negative story.
- Negative, judgmental body language generates mistrust and discourages patients from following the prescribed regimen.
- The best way to overcome negative comments about one's practice is to listen and find ways to improve.

Chapter 15
Endowment Effect
Noah Z. Feldman

The **Endowment Effect** is the preference for items that you already own, or are *endowed* with. Thus, if I were to first give you a coffee mug and then asked you if you wanted to trade it in for a pen of objectively equal value, you likely wouldn't accept the trade. On the other hand, if I were to first give you the pen, and then offered to trade it for the coffee mug, you, again, would hold on to the item you already have. The mental focus on positive factors of the item you already have—such as an attractive logo on the mug in the former case or the writing ability of the pen—powers the Endowment Effect; the Endowment Effect is a bias that causes irrational decisions to be made based off the wholly irrelevant factor of which item you started with.

Mathematically, the Endowment Effect occurs whenever the price at which someone will buy an item (WTP) is less than the price at which someone will accept to give up the item (WTA); when rational economic theory would propose that they are equal. This fairly basic rule of economic thought, that every item has a specific value for us at any point in time, is frequently broken.

Background and History
The Endowment Effect itself was discovered in the late 1960's,[100] but was only later coined by the economist Richard Thaler in 1980. Because it was tied together with loss aversion

for so long, the first experiments that directly studied the Endowment Effect didn't come about until the early 2000's. A study of college students' willingness to part with basketball tickets gives perhaps the clearest example of the Endowment Effect.[101] Duke University has intensely popular basketball games; these games are so popular that to get a ticket students need to camp-out by the box-office for several days. Even then there are more buyers than tickets, so the university instituted a lottery for those who had camped. The students who had camped were surveyed to determine for how much those who had won a ticket would be willing to sell it (WTA) and for how much those that didn't win one would pay to buy one (WTP). The results pointed to a staggeringly huge amount of the Endowment Effect: those who had won the tickets would need about $1,500 to sell, while those who hadn't won would only pay up to $150 to buy.

Examples and Analysis
The Endowment Effect applies very often, and the clearest examples come when people are making decisions between two similar items. This effect allows appliance stores to offer excellent return policies. Beyond the hassle of physically returning the appliance, people prefer the appliance they already own (i.e. are endowed with), so they keep it even if there is another one that would suit them better. The Endowment Effect also explains how people become attached to their randomly assigned seats in a football stadium or gifts in a white elephant game: Once they get an item, they value it more highly than the alternatives, even though their assignment to that item was random.

The Endowment Effect bias inverts when deciding between negative choices (taking out the trash versus doing the dishes, for example) because people value the option they currently have more negatively. If you have the job of doing the dishes and then are given the option to take out the trash instead, you are more likely to choose the latter than if you had been given a straight choice between the two. This is a repulsion to the endowed item rather than a standard attraction seen before. Also the Endowment Effect tends to disappear when the choice is between two objects with similar qualities. This means that if you are deciding between two cars — for example, a 50,000 miler that you have owned for 4 years and a new car of the same model — the endowment won't be pushing you toward the old one; this is because they share the same qualities, just in different amounts. Similarly, if you currently have a low quality generic pen and someone offers you a slightly higher quality generic pen, you will pick the higher quality pen even if you wouldn't have traded for a mug with a value equal to that of the higher value, second pen.

An explanation for the Endowment Effect is one of salience. People emphasize the facets of the object they have, so, if we look at the example at the top of this chapter, people with pens value writing abilities more highly (when considering the issue) and people with mugs value the ability to hold coffee highly. This inflation also works in the negative case. People with trash duty overemphasize the stench and people with the job of doing the dishes emphasize the resulting drying and irritation of their skin. This also explains why the Endowment Effect ceases for objects of the same type:

characteristics are inflated, so when objects share similar characteristics there is no net relative effect.[33] Other explanations of the Endowment Effect exist (you might trust the endowed item more, or transaction costs might be prohibitive) but they fall outside the realm of behavioral economics.

Applications in Medicine
Imagine that there are two medications: drugs A and B. You have been prescribing drug A for a long time; it works fairly well, but doesn't manage to clear up the problem completely. Drug B, on the other hand, is new, and you're deciding whether you want to switch your patients to it. Drug B is marginally more effective most of the time, but it does come with a few significant side effects. Because of the Endowment Effect, you may tend to inflate the positive aspect of drug A (lack of side effects) and chose to stick with it.

This also works from a patient's point of view. Say that a patient is deciding between two medications. He can't take both because they react negatively when combined. One medication treats a congenital skin condition and the other helps keeps his aging joints healthy. Because the skin condition is less of a nuisance than maladjusted joints, the patient would normally select the latter. But since he's been taking the skin medication for a while, the Endowment Effect may kick in and cause the patient to stick to the medication they are currently using. It might fall in the doctor's purview to give a little kick towards the second medication, if only to reduce the existing tendency to stick with the status quo.

But decisions between choices in the medical world are not limited to medicines. Medical administrators scheduling appointment slots and office managers rearranging work schedules or locations (for their own arcane machinations) are often left in the unenviable position of asking people to move from their regular locations, and regularly have to overcome the Endowment Effect to accomplish this. By phrasing their request as a choice between equal options (you can be at desk A or B, but I prefer B) rather than movement from the current condition (you can go from desk A to desk B, and I'd prefer you do) they can reduce this effect and make their jobs that much easier.

Quick Tips

- People become attached to items they own, and are usually unwilling to exchange them for other items of equal value.
- People also become more averse to negative situations they are endowed with, and usually prefer to switch to a less familiar situation of equal negative value.
- Endowment effects may reduce patients' willingness to switch to a different treatment.

Chapter 16
Meaning
Aleksandra Florek, Scott A. Davis, Steven R. Feldman

Meaning is a characteristic of human thinking that acts as a hidden, powerful motivational driver of productivity and effort. Meaningful work is defined as understanding one's sense of purpose and/or receiving acknowledgement or reward for one's efforts. When given the meaning of an action or task, individuals tend to perform with higher efficacy. In the book *The Outliers: The True Story of Success,* author Malcolm Gladwell explains that in order for one's work to be gratifying and fulfilling, it has to contain the following principles: autonomy, complexity, and a connection between effort and reward.[102] Many people would be happier earning $75,000 working as an architect than earning $100,000 working as a tollbooth operator.[102] Monetary reward alone does not offer long term satisfaction; it is the complexity of the work, daily appreciation, and recognition that provide gratification and drive productivity.

Background and History
The effects of meaning can be seen in motivation to learn a foreign language. Have you ever tried to learn a foreign language by memorizing lists of vocabulary words, grammar rules, and so on? For those who study a foreign language purely because it is an academic requirement, learning a language can be drudgery. For people who plan to use the language, perhaps for a trip to a foreign country, there is a much greater sense of purpose, realizing that not knowing

certain words can lead to serious consequences – ranging from a social faux pas to getting run over because you didn't understand a road sign. Moreover, the sense of appreciation you feel from people in the foreign country for your having tried to learn some of their language gives you further motivation to learn.

When presented with meaning, people tend to behave differently from what is predicted by a rational choice, utility maximizing model in which monetary payment would be the sole driving force of human productivity. Because people are heavily driven by non-monetary gratification, the standard, rational, utility maximizing model can fail if meaningfulness is not considered part of the utility that is maximized.

In regard to some life experiences, human beings often do not have an innate sense of whether an experience or task is good or bad. Undeniably there are many exceptions to this rule, for instance, losing a loved one is viewed as a uniformly negative experience. However, generally, it is possible for an incidental experience to be either desired or feared by a person, depending on its context and presentation. By developing the proper mindset, people may view a negative situation and be able to transform it into a positive experience. "There is nothing either good or bad," said Shakespeare, "but thinking makes it so."

Creating a cognitive bias can be used to increase productivity in the work place. By providing appreciation and appraisal to simple, monotonous, and repetitive labor, we may increase productivity and improve the final outcome. Meaningful work can be defined as receiving acknowledgment for one's efforts. William James, an American philosopher and psychologist who was also trained as a physician, once said, "The deepest principle in human nature is the craving to be appreciated." By providing sincere, honest appreciation and encouragement to our coworkers, superiors, and/or patients, we may help to paint negative or neutral tasks as positive experiences and thus create miracles on a daily basis! For example, at the end of a presentation or a lecture, we may dedicate the last slide to thank sincerely the specific people who were also involved in the work as well as even include their photograph. Such praise and appreciation will only create further incentive to work harder and place greater drive and effort into the work. The appreciation has to be sincere and come from the heart in order to provide fruitful results; otherwise, the meaning of the appraisal would be worthless. Appreciation is a neglected skill, yet if applied, it may tremendously increase not only productivity in the marketplace but patient adherence as well.

Examples and Analysis

A series of behavioral experiments in which subjects built Lego Bionicle robots demonstrated the value of meaning in task performance.[103] Investigators paid subjects to build the models, paying a diminishing rate for each additional Lego model built. Subjects were randomized into two work groups: Meaningful and Sisyphean. Under the "Meaningful" condition, subjects built multiple copies of Lego models, during which they were allowed to accumulate the finished models and thus witness the outcome of their effort. Under the "Sisyphean" condition, while the subjects were working on the subsequent Bionicle robot, the researchers took apart their previous newly built Lego creation, giving the subject the pieces to rebuild. This condition was named for the Greek myth of Sisyphus, who is condemned by gods to forever roll a rock up to the top of a mountain, only to have the rock roll back down to the bottom every time he reaches the top. The gods had thought that there was no worse punishment than repetitive, futile labor.[103]

In the "Meaningful" condition, subjects who were able to watch their finished models accumulate made more models (11 compared to 7) and required lower monetary payment for the task compared to the group in the "Sisyphean" condition. The result would suggest that there is something particularly demotivating when performing cyclical actions without a purpose. The researchers described meaningful work as providing a sense of purpose and/or acknowledgment. The authors proposed that a sense of meaning was a hidden motivational driver of productivity and served as a supplemental reward for a desired behavior. The results of this experiment show that payment is not necessarily the sole driver for motivation and productivity, but instead the emotional value of meaning of one's labor also drives motivation.[103]

In another experiment, college students were asked to find sets of repeated letters on a sheet of paper. The study divided the students into three subgroups.[103] A "supervisor" reviewed the work of the first group of the students as soon as it was turned in. Second group of students was told in advance that their work would be collected but not reviewed, and the third one watched as their papers were shredded immediately upon completion. Each of the students was paid 55 cents for completing the first sheet, and five cents less for each sheet thereafter. The participants were also informed that they may stop working at any point. The research team found that people whose work was reviewed and acknowledged by the "supervisor" were willing to do more work for less pay than those whose work was ignored or shredded. As for the other two groups, statistically speaking, ignoring the performance of people had almost the same effect as destroying the final product. It seems as though people are more productive when they feel a sense of purpose and see the fruits of their accomplishments.[103]

Another study assessed how context can affect perceptions of the value of an experience.[19] In one study participants were randomly assigned to two groups: the first group was asked whether they would be willing to receive US$2 to listen to a professor recite Walt Whitman poetry; the second group was asked whether they would be willing to pay US$2 to listen to the same poetry recital. After answering the initial question, the respondents were then asked if they would be willing to attend the recital for free. Students in the first group (who had been asked if they were willing to be paid to listen to the recital) were less likely than the students in the second group (students who had been asked if they would pay to attend the recital) to attend for free. Merely asking the students a question about willingness to pay or be paid had a substantial effect on how they perceived the value of the recital. This experiment showed that people's perception of an experience can vary from desired to avoided, depending on the context. In other words, the value of work or labor may be altered or molded by the context of the particular situations.[19] As our patients have to pay for their medications as well as for the office visits, it may be safe to say that their value of the consultations and visits is placed higher than if they were to receive free medication and not have to pay for their visits.

Voter turnout can also be improved by influencing the meaning that citizens attribute to voting. In *The Behavioral Foundations of Public Policy*, authors explained that voter mobilization efforts are more successful when they are communicated through more personal media, for example face-to-face advertising. Voting may mean to some people an avenue to express one's personal and social identity, and similarly to the previous studies, can be influenced by actions occurring before and after the moment of voting.[104]

Blood donations are another instance illustrating that meaning and context of situations can drive people to "donate" their time and resources to the greater need of society. The thought of helping another human being and potentially saving a life supersedes the lack of monetary compensation. Individuals often donate to various charities because they would like to feel appreciated by providing unselfish, marvelous acts. Many may argue that philanthropists do not donate in order to truly help others but do so in order to feel important, appreciated, and respected. Long distance runners can also represent an example of how meaning alters the perception of reality. Why would anyone want to complete a grueling 26 mile run or even a 5 k race? Perhaps they are running for a race where money is donated for a cure, such as for psoriasis or breast cancer. There are certain organizations which guarantee that more money is donated to the medical research depending on the amount of completed miles. This incentive then serves to drive the runners to have longer endurance, in order to provide more resources to the populations in need. The race numbers that people collect may be worth a miniscule amount, however, they often represent to the runner the accomplishment of completing the race. Society is often driven by outcomes, and being able to see the accomplishment may create a sense of pride and motivate people to work. *The Secret,* by Rhonda Byrne, describes creating a vision board of goals and dreams in life and hanging it up in the house. Visualizing the goal or outcome creates a meaning to people to pursue daily struggle; it gives them hope that their hard work will have an end result if only they will persevere.

Meaning makes a significant contribution to people's perceptions of reality. Although standard economic theory focuses on quantitative measures of value, such as monetary compensation, humans are also affected by the concealed meaning of what they do. People look for purpose and find value in making an impact. People are willing to perform tedious tasks, even for little pay, as long as they consider the work meaningful or are recognized for their contributions. A long journey or task is worth enduring when people know that when it is completed they are contributing to the greater good or if there is a worthwhile positive outcome at the finish line. We care about reaching a peak, and when we know that there is a meaning to our work, we are more willing to endure the struggle in order to each this peak.

Applications in Medicine

We can change perspective and change meaning to affect the way people accept a situation. Cancer patients may view chemotherapy as poison if they are viewing it in the context of side effects, but if it is emphasized as a special medicine created to treat them, these patients may be more eager to attend their chemotherapy sessions. They will be willing to endure the side effects if it implies that they will live a longer or better life than with the disease.

Perhaps one of the greatest responsibilities that we as physicians can do is to provide recognition and encouragement of the entire healthcare team. Charles Schwab has phrased beautifully a way to flourish the ambitions of people, "I consider my ability to arouse enthusiasm among my people the greatest asset I possess, and the way to develop the best that is in a person is by appreciation and encouragement. There is nothing else that so kills the ambitions of a person as criticism from superiors. I never criticize anyone. I believe in giving a person incentive to work. So I am anxious to praise but loath to find fault. If I like anything, I am hearty in my appreciation and lavish in my praise."[105] As physicians, the main coordinators of care, we should provide constant appreciation and recognition to our coworkers, including front desk administrators, marketing coordinators, drug representatives, nurses, lab technicians, volunteers in the office, and of course, our patients. For example, we should take action and compliment our patients on their lifestyle changes, "I noticed that you have lost weight, quit smoking and drinking alcohol, I would like to congratulate you and point out that your health is much better now that you have undertaken these lifestyle measures."

We are often baffled by how many of our patients with chronic conditions do not take their medications as prescribed. By increasing patient adherence, we can ensure that optimal care is provided for our patients. Often, patients do not feel the need to take medications because they believe it has little or no effect on their disease. Noncompliance is often the highest when symptoms are not immediately experienced. It is crucial that we identify the psychological barriers that patients have that prevent patients from adhering to their treatment regimen. Perhaps looking at a bottle of pills reminds them that they are ill. Perhaps the meaning of a pill bottle is disease, and as long as they are symptom-free, they choose to ignore the prescription. Perhaps the meaning of words themselves changes the outlook of the words. If we mention compliance, we imply that patients are passive actors in the management of their conditions. "Adherence," according to the World Health Organization, implies something very different from "compliance": that doctors and patients team up to actively engage in maintaining their health.[106, 107]

Charity donation has also been used as an incentive to adhere to the medication regimen. In particular, patients would receive a cell phone reminder that a portion of their prescription price, as little as 5 cents, would be donated to an assigned charity, for example AIDS United or the American Diabetes Association.[108] Even the smallest acknowledgement increases the willingness to participate in patient-physician relationship. We should allow patients to feel a sense of completion and ensure that a job well done is acknowledged. It is about the fact that the fruits of one's labor have some kind of survival beyond their pure existence. That is, somebody else would appreciate it, benefit from it; and appreciate the person who created it. All these things play a huge role in how we view our own labor.

Fear alters patients' perception of reality; thus our job as physicians is to change this perception. If someone is afraid of pain or blood we need to change their perception of these entities in order to make them willing to go through treatment. Making a child patient feel like a superhero for undergoing diagnostic procedures is a commonly applied technique by nurses. If children are to undergo a scan, such as an MRI, for example, we can reframe it as great fun by telling them they are going into a spaceship.[109] Giving them a certificate of completion after finishing treatment like chemotherapy or radiation gives them a sensation of success.

As Dan Ariely has stated in his book, "Maybe we feel meaning only when we deal with something bigger. Perhaps we hope that someone else, especially someone important to us, will ascribe value to what we've produced? Maybe we need the illusion that our work might one day matter to many people. That it might be of some value in the big, broad world out there [...]? Most likely it is all of these. But fundamentally, I think that almost any aspect of meaning [...] can be sufficient to drive our behavior. As long as we are doing something that is somewhat connected to our self-image, it can fuel our motivation and get us to work much harder."[21]

Realizing that many of our patients are very spiritual, we may increase adherence of these patients by painting a picture of their body as a sacred temple, which should be respected and cherished. After all, we were given only one body and irreversible damage may be done if not appropriately respected. When we present this image of a sacred temple to our patients, we will potentially induce greater adherence to medications. Perhaps we may even show some of the patients computerized images of what they will look like or what they will feel like if they do not follow a proper diet, exercise, and take their medications on a regular basis.

Quick Tips

- Making work meaningful with recognition and appreciation can greatly improve productivity in our offices.
- Some experiences can be viewed as either tedious or exciting, depending on how they are presented.
- Paying close attention to the meaning that the patient ascribes to treatment, and possibly adding an altruistic component, can improve motivation and adherence.

Chapter 17
Belief Bias
Asmaa Al-Kadhi, Scott A. Davis, and Steven R. Feldman

Belief bias is the tendency to judge the strength of arguments based on the plausibility of their conclusion rather than how strongly they support that conclusion. This bias can underlie faulty beliefs patients hold about disease and its treatment.

Background and History
In reasoning, an argument can be invalid while its conclusion is true, and an argument can be valid even if its conclusion is not true, if it is built on false premises. An argument's validity can be established using formal logic. A logical (valid) argument is guaranteed by laws of formal logic to be true if its premises are true. An illogical argument might coincidentally have a true conclusion, but its truth is not guaranteed by any logical principles. Belief bias creeps in when an invalid argument with a false conclusion is incorrectly thought to be valid because of a preconceived belief in the truth of the conclusion.

In three experiments by Evans, Barston and Pollard[110], 10% of participants accepted invalid conclusions to unbelievable arguments, while 71% of participants accepted invalid conclusions to believable arguments, suggesting that participants base their responses on belief rather than logical necessity.[111] For example, few participants endorsed the validity of the argument, "All fish are phylones (a made-up category). All phylones are trout. Therefore, all fish are trout." However, many participants said the following argument was valid: "All fish are phylones. All phylones are trout. Therefore, all trout are fish."[111] Presumably, the participants believed that all trout are fish, but did not believe that all fish are trout, so they did not realize that only the first argument was logically sound (although it may have faulty premises).

Subjects tend to examine the conclusion and, if it is believable, simply accept it without further ado and without even looking at the argument. On the other hand, if the conclusion is unbelievable, they will then attempt to analyze the logic of the problem to see if the conclusion is valid or not. Even scientists are not immune to belief bias. A scientific paper with poor methods but a conventional conclusion may be more likely to get accepted for publication than one with excellent methods that challenges an entrenched dogma.

Examples and Analysis

Belief bias arises due to a conflict occurring between belief and logical reasoning.[112] In logical reasoning, the conclusion is drawn from two given premises; a major premise (often a general statement) and a minor premise (a more specific instance) are used to draw a conclusion.[113] Each of the premises has one word in common with the conclusion. Examples:

- Major premise: All humans are mortal.
- Minor premise: Socrates is human.
- Conclusion: Socrates is mortal.

In this example the major premise shares *mortal* with the conclusion while the minor premise shares *Socrates*.

The above example is correct and its conclusion is valid; it is a correct application of a true logical principle. The example below might seem to make sense, but actually upon close examination, it is invalid:

- Major premise: All medical students participate in research.
- Minor premise: John participates in research.
- Conclusion: Therefore John is a medical student.

In this example all the premises are right, but the form of the argument is illogical and thus invalid. The form of the argument is "all A's do B; C does B; therefore C is an A," which is an example of a logical flaw called the converse error. Although full discussion of logic errors is beyond the scope of this book, this argument subtly differs from the argument "all A's do B; C is an A; therefore C does B," which is logical and valid. The human brain has to be trained in formal logic to recognize the error, and since most people are not trained in formal logic, they fall back on simpler modes of thinking. Their preconceived notions about the plausibility of the conclusion influence their judgment of the validity of the argument, resulting in a belief bias.

In general, people will tend to discard conclusions that do not fit in with their belief schemes, even though these conclusions may be perfectly logical and arguably possible. This is true when people ignore the premises and focus solely on the conclusions being drawn; therefore belief bias surfaces when the given conclusion does not fit with the person's beliefs and knowledge.

Applications in Medicine

An example of a belief bias occurred at a community clinic, when a patient with Herpes Zoster (shingles) of the ophthalmic branch of the trigeminal nerve mentioned to the doctor that he is applying honey on all the vesicles, believing that it would help to make the healing process faster. The provider tried to explain that the honey is processed honey and there is a difference between table honey and medical-grade honey;[114] the processed one which is in the grocery stores may lead to an opposite effect. The patient argued that the ancient Egyptians used honey to cure wounds and he has a belief in natural remedies. A few days passed and the patient came back complaining of yellowish crusted non-healing vesicles with secondary bacterial skin infection.

Back to our belief bias:
- Major premise: Honey has been used to cure skin lesions (shingles is a skin lesion) by ancient Egyptians.
- Minor premise: The product sold in the grocery store is honey.
- Conclusion: The product sold in the grocery store will cure shingles.

Here the structure of the argument appears logical, parallel to the "Socrates is mortal" example. However, the word "honey" refers to natural honey in the major premise and processed honey in the minor premise, making the argument invalid. Since the patient has a strong belief in natural remedies, he easily overlooks this subtle error and accepts an invalid argument that confirms his pre-existing belief.

Background knowledge is thought to obstruct the reasoning process by altering the way the premises are interpreted, that is, by making logically unnecessary conclusions appear necessary.[115] Markovits and Nantel suggested the belief-bias effect would be less evident if subjects were asked to produce their own conclusions than if asked to evaluate the validity of a presented conclusion.[116] Therefore it's better to ask about the patient's belief. Why is the patient thinking that a certain medication will work while others will not?

In drawing a conclusion, people use two processes: the first involves the generation of a conclusion (or conclusions) by a process of reasoning; the second involves a process of evaluation during which extra-logical factors (factors outside the realm of logic and reasoning) such as belief might enter in.[116] Therefore when discussing different modalities of medications or surgical procedures with the patient, in order to decrease this biasing effect, we must take in consideration the interference of extra-logical factors such as beliefs, interference from family members and friends and financial ability; all those resources might affect the patient's conclusion. When feasible, we might just want to accept that the bias is present and use framing (see Chapter 5) to our advantage. For example, when prescribing a vitamin D cream for psoriasis, we can emphasize that it is an "all natural" vitamin D product.

It's advisable to listen tentatively to the patients, address their beliefs seriously and when necessary, be ready to explain why their conclusion is invalid in a caring, nonthreatening way.

Quick Tips

- People tend to judge arguments by the believability of their conclusions rather than whether they are logical.
- Ask about a patient's reasoning process to uncover hidden biases that might influence their choice of treatment.
- Framing a treatment in a way that fits with the patient's pre-existing beliefs is one way to avoid negative reactions from belief bias.

Chapter 18
Hedonic Treadmill
Irma M. Richardson, Scott A. Davis, and Steven R. Feldman

The **hedonic treadmill** is the term used to describe the tendency for people's happiness to quickly adjust to changes in circumstances. This theory explains that, as a person makes more money, expectation and desires rise in tandem and therefore no permanent gain in happiness results. Losses and gains in finances may temporarily affect how happy one is, but most people will return to their set point of normal level of happiness.

Over time psychologists have changed the term to "hedonic adaptation", a phenomenon in which people adapt to changes, whether good or bad, to maintain stable happiness.[117] This can include not only financial changes, but also changes in other areas such as health and relationships.

Background
The term hedonic treadmill began in 1971 by Brickman and Campbell in the article "Hedonic Relativism and Planning the Good Society".[118] The general concept is even though external forces are continually changing in an individual's life, happiness is relatively constant.

Examples
The hedonic treadmill phenomenon does appear to lend credence to the expression "Money can't buy happiness." For most people the pursuit of happiness is just as satisfying as

actually finding it. Brickman et al. concluded that lottery winners were not happier than nonwinners and that people with paraplegia were not substantially less happy than those who can walk.[117] People continue to pursue happiness because they incorrectly believe that greater happiness lies just around the corner in the next goal accomplished, the next social relationship obtained, or the next problem solved.[117] Suh, Diener, and Fujita found that good and bad life events affected happiness only if they occurred in the past two months. They also found people tend to recover from both positive and negative life events.[119]

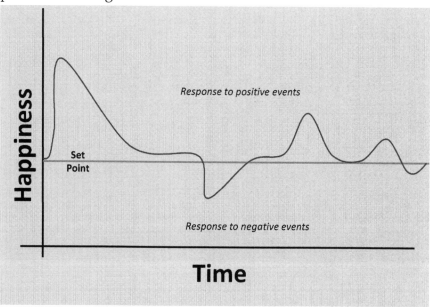

Figure 1. Happiness adjusts to both positive and negative events over time. After a positive event such as winning the lottery, it initially rises, but eventually the person adapts and happiness falls back to the set point. Similarly, after a negative event such as a major injury, happiness drops but eventually rises back to the set point.

Application to Medicine

Several cross-sectional studies have explored the outcomes of positive or negative medical events. In patients that had surgery for breast cancer, 1 to 60 months after surgery for breast cancer, the majority of patients reported that their lives had been altered for the better.[120] People who are blind do not differ in happiness from those who are able to see.[121] Individuals with spinal cord injuries report strong negative emotions one week after their crippling accidents, yet two months later, happiness was their strongest emotion.[122]

One benefit of this characteristic of human psychology is that the impact of chronic disease on quality of life tends to lessen over time as patients get used to their condition. On the other hand, we should also expect that patients' joy in improving their condition or recovering from illness is also likely to be ephemeral. Cosmetic surgery is an elective procedure to enhance a person's appearance. Cosmetic surgery is often used as an option to regain a youthful appearance, build self-esteem, or become beautiful according to society's standards. There is apparent happiness following a successful surgery. However, changing the outward appearance is not likely to change the mental happiness set point; it is not clear how long changes in happiness will last.

Hedonic adaptation can affect adherence behavior. A patient who improved greatly may at first be very happy, but over time they may begin to complain that the medication is "no longer working".[123, 124] In diseases that are not curable, the patient may suddenly realize that they will have to take the medication for the rest of their life, which may seem daunting.

For this type of patient, we may have to remind them how bad they felt in the past and how much they would lose by going back to a worse disease state. If it is possible to reduce the frequency or intensity of the regimen, and we suggest this option, the patient may feel we've read their mind. Although this action may seem trivial, many patients feel very anxious or guilty about having defied medical advice by using the medication less.[56] Therefore, as soon as we put our stamp of approval on the change in regimen, the patient may breathe a huge sigh of relief.

Understanding the hedonic treadmill may help us understand the best ways to interact with changes in our health care system. A sudden negative change of large magnitude may leave us feeling down, but we will quickly adapt. A continuous series of minor traumas and irritations with electronic medical records and new bureaucratic hassles is likely to have a greater impact on our psyche. To the extent that we have control over implementing changes in our own practices and with our staff, it may be best to bite the bullet and make large changes once, rather than making many smaller changes over time.

Most importantly, though, we are who are in the health care profession should realize that we are living in the greatest time in human history. With our cars, airplanes, central heating and air conditioning, air & food quality, cell phones, iPods, access to information over the Internet, and indoor plumbing, we live better than most of the kings and queens in human history. If we can keep in mind that our worst days are better than the best days of most of the people who have ever lived, perhaps we can force our conscious minds to see past the hedonic treadmill and find continuous joy in the lives we lead.

Quick Tips

- Happiness tends to return to the original set point over time, rather than staying up or down after an event.
- Patients who feel that their medication is "no longer working" may be experiencing the adjustment back to normal after a high point.
- Over the long run, a single large negative event may be preferable to a succession of smaller negative events.

Chapter 19
The Easterlin Paradox
Brandy H. Sullivan, Scott A. Davis, and Steven R. Feldman

Above a certain point, increases in income do not increase an individual's happiness, a phenomenon termed the Easterlin Paradox [125]. While happiness (or social welfare) is a by-product of economic welfare, happiness is not solely derived from the reward of prosperity or an increase in wealth (Figure 1)[126]. Happiness is a social outcome that is immensely difficult to standardize as it becomes a fluctuating descriptor that is bound by the fortune or misfortune, emotion, hope, desires, and satisfaction of an individual.

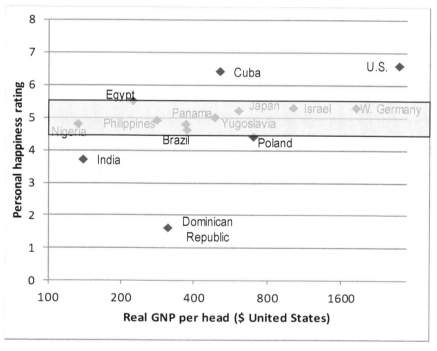

Figure 1: Personal happiness rating and GNP per head (in 1960 U.S. currency), 14 countries. [127] Reprinted by permission.

This article was published in *Nations and Households in Economic Growth: Essays in Honour of Moses Abramovitz*, edited by P.A. David and Melvin W. Reder. Copyright Elsevier, 1974.

Background & History

The Easterlin Paradox was originally described by Richard A. Easterlin in a chapter he wrote in 1974 entitled, "Does Economic Growth Improve the Human Lot? Some Empirical Evidence".[126] The data employed are gathered from surveys assessing the self-reporters' subjective happiness. There are two types of data gathered from this experiment. The first data collected were the responses to a Gallup-poll-type or opinion poll survey in which through a series of questions the opinions of a population are assessed and generalizations are made through statistical interpretation of the data. These questions included: "In general, how happy would you say you are-- very happy, fairly happy, or not very happy?"; and if they could describe what happiness means to them in their own words. As income increased, happiness increased up to a point (about $40,000 in today's dollars) and then leveled off (Figure 2). Also, happiness did not increase over time despite rising incomes. These results suggested that once certain basic needs were satisfied, happiness did not rise any further with increasing income, most likely because people above a modest level of income based their happiness on comparison with a reference group. Since richer people had a wealthier reference group, they did not feel any better off than middle-class people who had a middle-class reference group.

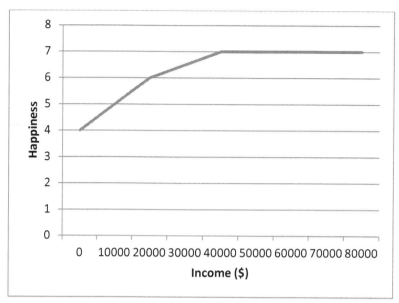

Figure 2. Happiness increases with income only up to a certain point. Once basic needs are satisfied, increased income is not associated with increased happiness.

"The Pattern of Human Concerns" study used data from 14 countries with the objective of determining both national and personal aspirations; for 10 out of the 14 countries, there was no direct correlation between personal happiness and an increase in national capital within or between countries (Table 1). [127]

Country (Date)	# groups	Rating of lowest status group	Rating of highest status group	Difference	N
United States (1959)	5	6.0	7.1	1.1	1549
Cuba (1960)	3	6.2	6.7	0.5	992
Israel (1961-62)	3	4.0	6.5	2.5	1170
West Germany (1957)	3	4.9	6.2	1.3	480
Japan (1962)	3	4.3	5.8	1.5	972
Yugoslavia (1962)	4	4.3	6.0	1.7	1523
Philippines (1959)	4	4.1	6.2	2.1	500
Panama (1962)	2	4.3	6.0	1.7	642
Nigeria (1962-63)	2	4.7	5.8	1.1	1200
Brazil (1960-61)	5	3.9	7.3	3.4	2168
Poland (1962)	5	3.7	4.9	1.2	1464
India (1962)	4	3.0	4.9	1.9	2366
Dominican Republic (1962)	2	1.4	4.3	2.9	814
Average		4.2	6.0	1.8	

Table 1: Personal happiness rating for lowest and highest social groups, 13 countries. [127] Reprinted by permission. This article was published in *Nations and Households in Economic Growth: Essays in Honour of Moses Abramovitz*, edited by P.A. David and Melvin W. Reder. Copyright Elsevier, 1974.

Examples and Analysis

Happiness is determined by an individual's social experience, current and past, not simply by income or wealth. For example, a single mother of three living in the inner-city has a very different point of reference or context from which she draws than a married mother of three living in a suburban neighborhood in the same state. Their context — neighborhood or social environment — creates benchmarks for happiness different for each woman. Perhaps, for the single mother of three, happiness is being able to supply a sufficient amount of food for each child each day while maintaining the home and paying all bills on time. Whereas the married mother of three, happiness may be defined as being able to maintain the home to the higher standards of her community, to be as a stay-at-home wife, to drive a Lexus SUV like her neighbors. Humans are constructed to view happiness and social situations relative to reference points.

While Easterlin's findings suggest that monetary goals cannot consistently improve human happiness, there are some strategies to follow to increase happiness. Experiences tend to result in more happiness than possessions.[128] We quickly adjust our reference points and become accustomed to having the possessions, while the experiences are remembered better with the passage of time (Figure 3a; see also Chapter 24, Rosy Retrospection). This is the opposite of what rational choice theory would predict, as a rational animal would no longer feel any pleasure from an experience after it had ended, but would continue to feel pleasure from a possession for as long as they were able to use it (Figure 3b).

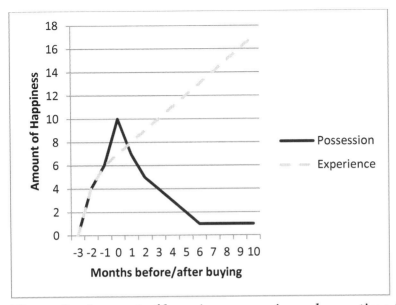

Figure 3a. Amount of happiness experienced over time from a possession vs. an experience. In both cases, people begin to feel pleasure before the purchase by anticipating the purchase. However, the pleasure from the experience may continue to rise after the experience ends, due to rosy retrospection. On the other hand, people quickly adjust to having the possession, so the pleasure attached to it declines rapidly.

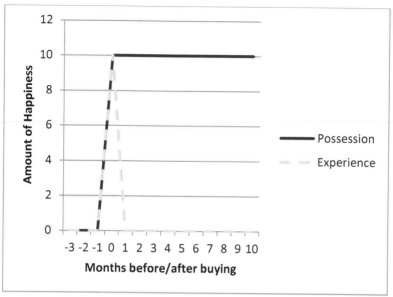

Figure 3b. In contrast, a rational actor model would predict that a rational animal would feel pleasure only during the experience itself, whereas they would continue to feel equal amounts of pleasure for as long as they used the possession. By spending more on experiences and less on possessions, we may increase our happiness without having to increase our income. Experiences shared with others, which create great shared memories, are likely to give even more happiness.

Applications in Medicine

For physicians, the Easterlin paradox may suggest that working more hours to increase our income is counterproductive. If we sacrifice vacation time with family to make more money, we will probably not increase our happiness, and may inadvertently send the message to our families that we do not care about them. Hospitals may be acting in a short-sighted fashion if they do not encourage their physicians to unplug for a while and invest in their families and relationships. The Easterlin paradox may also explain why many of us are happier to work in academic, military, or other health system (e.g. Kaiser) settings, even though we could make more money in private practice. Seeing patients all day every day might not be as much fun as seeing patients one day, then working with colleagues on a book on behavioral economics or a journal article the next day. With our employees, we may also find it more effective to incentivize them with more vacation or more flexibility in hours, rather than higher pay alone.

In this era of declining reimbursements, the Easterlin paradox may suggest strategies that we can use to maintain patient satisfaction while spending less money. "Patient-centered care" is the new buzzword, recommending that we stop spending money on interventions that patients do not care about, while emphasizing the human touch that they do care about. For example, some individuals may be happier when allowed to freely participate in religious activities that are significant to them, in addition to receiving appropriate treatment that does not hinder their religious expression; rather than receiving treatment, that while costly and more aggressive, would ultimately hinder their ability to engage their faith. In a study conducted over a five-year span (Sept 2002-Aug 2007) enlisting cancer patients from seven outpatient sites nationwide, Drs. Balboni and their team suggest that the end of life costs for cancer patients that held religion as a personal value, and were not supported in their religious practices by their healthcare team were significantly higher especially in minority and highly religious patient populations.[129]

Illness has a way of equalizing all are who impacted by it; illness does not discriminate according to wealth or the lack thereof. Using the example of terminal illness, such as cancer, happiness may be more defined by quality of life rather than quantity of days; and so, an individual may desire treatment options that would minimize the pain rather than curative measures. A terminally ill patient likely will desire a human touch and a few minutes of listening from a caring physician, which might mean more than a treatment costing thousands of dollars. According to Easterlin, the old adage holds true, money can't buy happiness. Because happiness is quite subjective for most individuals, money is not the only means of achieving happiness and there are many things we can do to improve patient satisfaction that cost nothing.

Quick Tips

- Happiness increases with increasing income only up to a modest amount, then levels off.
- Experiences generally give more happiness than possessions, as people quickly become accustomed to having the possessions.
- Giving up vacation time with family to earn more income is likely to be counterproductive.

PART IV

Misperceptions of Probability: How We Perceive Risks of Treatments

Chapter 20
Ostrich effect
Scott A. Davis, Asmaa Al-Kadhi, and Steven R. Feldman

The **ostrich effect** describes situations in which people ignore
an obvious negative situation and do not factor it into their
choices. It derives its name from the unforgettable (though
zoologically incorrect) image of an ostrich burying its head in
the sand to avoid danger. Investors, world leaders, physicians,
and patients are all susceptible to this bias, sometimes leading
to disastrous effects. Although this is a fertile area of research
in medicine that is still at an early stage, fortunately there are
many tactics we might use to get our patients' heads out of the
sand so they can make smart decisions.

Background and History
The ostrich effect was identified by Dan Galai and Orly Sade
in 2003.[130] They analyzed the difference between interest rates
on one-year bank deposits (similar to certificates of deposit
[CDs]) and one-year treasury bills in Israel. The treasury bills
offered higher interest rates, despite having no additional risk
and no penalty for early withdrawal as the bank deposits had.
Logically, it seemed that no one should choose the bank
deposits over the treasury bills, but many investors did. Galai
and Sade hypothesized that the treasury bills *seemed* riskier
because their prices were reported every day, unlike the bank
deposits. In support of the idea that the differences were due
to an ostrich effect, Galai and Sade found that the difference in
rates was larger in times of greater financial uncertainty.

Subsequently Niklas Karlsson, George Loewenstein, and

Duane Seppi extended the theory by analyzing the behavior of Scandinavian investors during good and bad markets, finding that investors checked the value of their investments 50 to 80% less often when the market was struggling.[131] They hypothesized that the ostrich effect was likely related to loss aversion, where people would prefer to ignore information about a potential loss for as long as possible to reduce the pain.

Although the behavioral economics usage of "ostrich effect" is of recent vintage, certainly there are many famous historical examples. British Prime Minister Neville Chamberlain appeased Hitler by letting Germany annex part of Czechoslovakia without a fight. Ignoring the long-term threat from Nazi Germany, Chamberlain proclaimed "peace in our time," but later found that Hitler could not be appeased. Soviet leader Joseph Stalin signed a non-aggression pact with Hitler and was caught unprepared when Hitler broke the treaty and invaded the Soviet Union. Some claim that Stalin retreated to his country home in disbelief for days following the invasion, although the story may have been a self-serving caricature created by Stalin's successor, Nikita Khrushchev.[132] It was Hitler's turn to play the ostrich when his troops were caught unprepared for the frigid Russian winter. These situations show that national leaders may be as prone to the ostrich effect as anyone else.

Examples and Analysis

The ostrich effect often takes the form of ignoring a known risk. This behavior can be adaptive if the risk is outweighed by a benefit inseparable from the risk. People whose lifelong dream was to have a beach house in California would lose a great deal of enjoyment if they constantly stressed about earthquakes, and Floridians tend to block out the nightmare scenario of a huge hurricane strike. Military recruiters are remarkably successful at getting enlistees to ignore the obvious risk of death in combat, and refocusing attention on the skills training, prestige, and financial benefits available to military personnel. For many recruits, the benefits do outweigh the risks, and in some years several civilian jobs have actually had a similar level of risk. Paradoxically, people who face a very low level of a risk (like hurricanes) may be quite worried, whereas those who face a higher level of risk are prone to the ostrich effect (Figure 1). This tendency, where the level of concern decreases when the risk increases, completely violates the assumptions of rational choice theory.

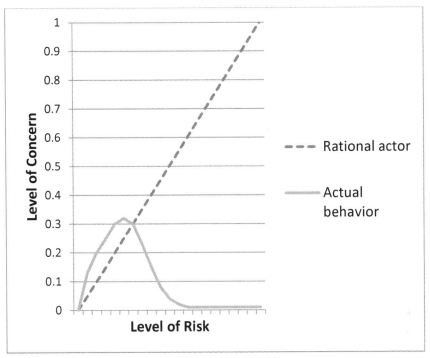

Figure 1. For a rational actor, the level of concern with a risk would increase linearly with the magnitude of the risk. For actual humans, the level of concern rises rapidly at low risks (see Chapter 21, Probability biases), but may drop to near zero as the risk increases into the "ostrich effect" zone.

Sometimes the results of the ostrich effect can be catastrophic, however, such as in the above examples from World War II. Fortunately, Britain had a democratic process that swept Chamberlain out of power immediately once it was clear his appeasement strategy had failed. In the other cases, an authoritarian leadership structure made it difficult to stop the ostrich-like leader from doing further damage. Even in democratic politics and business settings, a charismatic leader or clique can induce groupthink, where dissenters from an apparent consensus see their loyalty questioned. With groupthink, a group comes to a more extreme decision than most of the individuals in the group would have made on their own. When businesses have a cohesive leadership that limits debate to a narrow range of viewpoints, often rash decisions result. During the housing bubble, leaders of many banks silenced dissenters who thought that house prices might peak and crash because of mortgage lending to borrowers with poor credit.[133] When house prices did drop, foreclosures became rampant, and many banks failed or had to take emergency loans from the government. These examples may initially seem to have little relevance to us as physicians, but medical practice is often structured in a similar hierarchical fashion. Following a large number of highly publicized safety incidents, hospitals have reformed their practices to weaken the hierarchy, so that a nurse can call a time-out when concerned that a patient might be about to receive a wrong-site surgery.

Karlsson's stock market example would be a more equivocal instance of ostrich effect, with certain benefits but also potential negative consequences. It might have some benefits if it prevents panicked investors from selling all their stocks at the bottom, but overall it is considered irrational.[134] Generally financial advisors suggest avoiding negative consequences from the ostrich effect by setting up automatic transfers of the same amount every month to one's investment accounts. By automating the disciplined, stoic investing style that works best over the long term, this strategy may avoid panicked behavior and even call attention to the benefit of buying stocks at a bargain when the market is down.

Applications in Medicine

Patients are prone to ignore the consequences of all kinds of unhealthy behaviors, whether it is smoking, drinking, drug abuse, unhealthy eating, or nonadherence to an important medication. An example was a diabetic patient one of the authors saw. This patient came in with poor glycemic control and nonadherence to his medications and follow-up visits. When the physician explained the importance of foot care, emphasizing that the patient might get a peripheral neuropathy and wouldn't feel the injuries in his foot, the patient ignored the advice, arguing, "How will I not be able to feel the injury? I will see it!" After missing his next follow-up visit, by six months later he ended up with a foot ulcer and finally osteomyelitis. While one might think that inducing fear by showing the patient a disgusting picture of a foot ulcer would help, the theory of the ostrich effect suggests that employing fear would only intensify the patient's tendency to ignore the risks.

Although scientists are just beginning to explore how the ostrich effect might be mitigated in medicine, one key appears to be replacing negative and irrational thoughts with more positive, rational ones so that the patient might act more like the rational actor. Lund-Nielsen and colleagues studied breast cancer patients who had avoided treatment for a median of 24 months despite having a malignant breast cancer wound.[135] Common themes in their study included disbelief, shame, and finally relief after the patients finally overcame their initial motives for avoiding treatment (Table 1).

COMMENTS ABOUT DISBELIEF
• "If I had lied down to sleep at night and not woken up again, it would have been a relief because my [sick] siblings were such a burden for me. I had no time to look after myself. I was alone. I was forced to take responsibility because there was no one else." • "I saw my sisters go to the doctor for the same thing, and they all had operations, but it spread anyway later on. I thought that if I could avoid having the operation, I would be better off. So, I guess that I made a bit of a conscious decision not to go to the doctor because I couldn't let go of those other stories. I was the one who actually looked after them [sisters] while they were dying."

COMMENTS ABOUT SHAME
• "It kept getting worse and uglier to look at, and I did try to tell myself that if I went to the doctor now, it would look better than if I waited another 2 months – so do it! The shame came from the fact that if one was an intelligent, logical person, one would seek medical attention." • "I had to keep away from all of those whom I cared about. I had to build a wall around myself so that they didn't suspect anything. But they knew I was sick. I kept saying that I was not sick, and despite that, I went to the garage and vomit because I didn't want them to see. I felt like a hunted animal. It was really hard."

COMMENTS ABOUT RELIEF
• "Now we speak about it a lot with family and friends. Earlier on, it was very important to keep it a secret, but since it was discovered, it is important to speak openly about it. I don't hide the fact that I didn't bathe and that I had a few glasses too many of wine and gin – that came along with it all. It was great to come out of that deep secret place into the open – it was like being born again. It's a total relief."

Table 1. Quotes from patients in Lund-Nielsen's qualitative analysis, "An Avalanche of Ignoring", of comments from women who avoided treatment for breast cancer.[135]

Lund-Nielsen and colleagues conclude that we need "to assist the individual in correcting negative cognitions including the idea that health care may be harmful or dangerous and thereby install/restore approach behavior necessary for resolution of the problem and resumption of normal functioning."[135] Other strategies include trying to get the patient out of an environment where negative groupthink is common, and instead encouraging association with a more positive peer group. The financial examples considered in this chapter also suggest that automating positive behavior may reduce the tendency to make bad decisions during tough times. Just as investors should automate their saving behavior so that they invest even when the market is down, we should get patients into the habit of having an annual physical, ensuring that problems are detected at an early stage.

Perhaps the epitome of the ostrich effect is patients who have severe mistrust in physicians, medications, and the entire medical system. In the breast cancer example, the ostrich effect was characterized by depression, feeling overwhelmed, and self-blame. There is also a more defiant, even arrogant sort of mistrust that arises frequently. For example, many patients, especially men devoted to macho ideals, want to "just tough it out" to avoid admitting weakness or disability. Sometimes we can turn this maladaptive behavior on its head by challenging men, saying, "Most guys don't have what it takes to use this stuff. Do you think you can do it?" Advertisers of erectile dysfunction medications have had to learn this lesson to overcome some patients' reluctance to admit the need for medical help with their condition. A typical Viagra ad asks whether the viewer would attempt a risky golf shot over a pond on the 18th hole of a match, or lay up. Obviously the real man's choice is clear – he faces the problem head-on and does what has to be done. This example may be instructive for getting men to follow other health interventions as well.

Whether it manifests as feelings of incompetence or arrogance, the ostrich effect is closely linked to the psychological phenomenon of denial. Denial runs deep; as Cole and Bird write, "Through the process of denial and rationalization many smokers come to believe either that they are immune to the health risks or that the risks are too insignificant to bother with."[63] Overcoming denial is a major component of twelve-step programs like Alcoholics Anonymous. By having people admit to a group that they have an addiction, twelve-step programs establish a basis for using group pressure and accountability to overcome denial. In addition to the group as a whole, members usually have a sponsor who has gone through the same addiction and provides additional individualized support. We should be sure to make patients aware of support groups such as these in our area. If an appropriate twelve-step group is not available, we might ask whether the patient is interested in seeking help from a support group affiliated with the patient's place of worship. Although we as physicians are not in the business of promoting religion, patients who already have strong religious affiliations may welcome the participation of their religious communities in changing their unhealthy habits. In *The Power of Habit,* Charles Duhigg describes how pastor Rick Warren used home prayer groups to reinforce prosocial habits and build strong bonds that helped members through difficult times.[22]

Support groups for specific diseases — such as the Diabetes Advocacy Alliance, Asthma and Allergy Foundation of America, and National Psoriasis Foundation — also provide the benefit of absorbing the individual into a group that abides by common, social norms. In addition to other benefits we have discussed in prior chapters, these support groups normalize the experience of illness and its treatment. Each member learns that they are not the only one struggling with the disease (plus frustrating health system issues that might otherwise cause them to give up). Groups are typically not physician-led, so members feel like they can share experiences as peers without an authority figure in the room. Support group patients also may be offered frequent opportunities to participate in clinical trials, which have extra visits that enhance adherence to medications.[136] The clinical trials help normalize regular use of the medication, a habit that is self-sustaining once established.

For some patients, a strong tendency toward defiance of authority figures, or even the medical profession as a whole, may be the reason for poor adherence. These patients exhibit the ostrich effect because they are actually asserting their freedom of choice, which is more important to them than achieving good health (discussed in more detail in Chapter 11,

Submission and Resistance to Authority). Their brains may also be giving excessive weight to examples that downplay the risk of their behavior.[59] These patients may be pleasantly surprised when we meet them on their own turf, such as by asking what they like about drinking. Asking questions like, "Do you sometimes drink two or three six-packs on the weekend?" may make the patient more willing to admit to their actual level of drinking.[63] For patients who say they have taken several medications but still have active disease, we can empathize, "I bet these treatments have been very frustrating, haven't they?" The patient will think we've read their mind, but in fact patients are almost always frustrated by treatments if they still have active disease. After building rapport in this manner, we can ask what the patient sees as benefits of reducing the unhealthy behavior. This way, patients know they are not trying to modify their behavior to please us (extrinsic motivation), but are taking action to improve their own lives in ways that are intrinsically motivating and personally valued.

Quick Tips

- People often prefer to ignore negative situations, and sometimes their level of concern drops when the risk increases.
- We may have to help patients avoid groups that reinforce thoughts of hopelessness about their medical problems.
- For patients who are arrogant and don't want to admit that a medication will help, consider appealing to their self-concept that they take charge in other areas of life.

Chapter 21
Probability Biases
Scott A. Davis and Steven R. Feldman

Large numbers, especially those into the millions or billions, are difficult for the human brain to grasp. Very small fractions, such as 1/1,000,000, create similar problems. Modern life has greatly increased the frequency of situations where people must deal intelligently with very large numbers or very small probabilities. Today, we have to deal with human populations into the billions, government deficits stretching into the trillions of dollars, and also drugs with 1-in-1,000,000 risks, and Mega Millions lotteries with a 1-in-258,890,850 chance of winning.[137] **Probability biases** describe the human response to situations where either a risk is magnified greatly (**conservatism** or **regressive bias**), or different-sized risks are mistakenly treated as equivalent (**probability neglect**).

Background and History
Research showing that people tend to overrate the frequency of uncommon events and underrate the frequency of common events dates back at least to 1953, when Fred Attneave's study showed that subjects overrated the frequency of uncommon letters in a typical English text, while underrating the frequency of the most common letters.[138] Such studies suggested that an S-shaped curve described the psychological response to many phenomena, with overweighting of rare events and underweighting of frequent events. These discoveries laid the groundwork for further research in the 1990's and 2000's studying the reasons for the S-shaped

curvature of people's utility function (Figure 1).

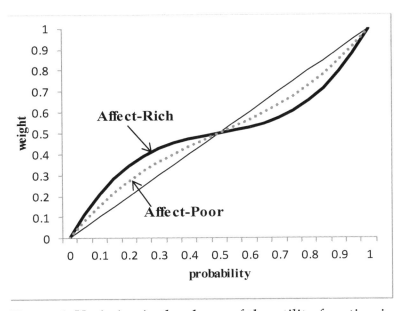

Figure 1. Variation in the shape of the utility function in affect-rich and affect-poor situations. Both have an S-shaped deviation from the rational actor's straight line, but the affect-rich situation shows the greatest deviation. (Rottenstreich and Hsee, *Psychological Science* Vol. 12 No. 3, pp. 185-190, Copyright © 2001 American Psychological Society, Reprinted by Permission of SAGE Publications.[139]) The S-shape of the curve shows that people place more weight than they should on events that have a very low probability and less weight then they should on events with a high probability. The shape of the curve is also related to the Certainty Effect described in Chapter 5. When people are certain, the weight they apply matches true probability; when there is uncertainty, the weight applied to the uncertainty is far greater than the true probability.

In 2001, Yuval Rottenstreich and Christopher Hsee found strong evidence that the S-shaped nature of the expected utility function was tied to the affective properties of the outcome. Affect-rich outcomes, such as those arousing strong emotion, showed large deviations from the straight line, while affect-poor outcomes showed much smaller deviations. For example, participants were willing to pay a median of $10 to avoid a 99% chance of a painful electric shock, and $7 to avoid a 1% chance of the same shock.[139] Participants were willing to pay more for a 1% chance of a prize when the prize was a $500 coupon for a European vacation (affect-rich) than when it was a $500 coupon for college tuition (affect-poor). However, they were willing to pay less for a 99% chance of the vacation prize than for a 99% chance of the tuition prize. In another study by Colin Camerer, cash prizes of thousands of dollars evoked more S-shaped utility curves than smaller cash prizes.[140] Large prizes gave rise to much larger emotional reactions, which led to an irrationally high willingness to pay for a small chance at the prize.

In 2002, Cass Sunstein identified probability neglect as the phenomenon in which, "when intense emotions are engaged, people tend to focus on the adverse outcome, not on its likelihood."[141] Sunstein cited a wide variety of examples ranging from overreaction to terrorism and inconsequential pollutants, to people paying the same amount for insurance against risks of different magnitudes. For example, people will pay more for flight insurance for losses resulting from terrorism, than for flight insurance for losses from all causes.[141] People will also pay about the same amount to insure against a 1/650 risk compared to a 1/68,000 risk,[142] although rational choice theory suggests that they should be willing to pay over 100 times more to insure against the higher risk. People also showed much greater willingness to take action in a "high-outrage" case (nuclear waste) than a "low-outrage" case (radon exposure), even when the risks were quantified as identical.[141] As in the case where people assert that a pound of lead is heavier than a pound of feathers, the emotional content of the mental imagery available to people far outweighs the statistics, which would be the sole basis for the decision by a rational actor.

Examples and Analysis

When faced with the possibility of an unlikely outcome, there is a common tendency to overestimate the risk of that outcome happening. If the risk is simply stated as, "there is a chance of X happening," without further characterizing how much chance, people may tend to assume that it is an equal (50-50) chance. Thus if there is a small risk of a very bad outcome, such as death or cancer, people may catastrophize and behave as if there is a 50-50 risk. If the risk is first stated without any detail, and only later quantified exactly, people might have already chosen 50-50 as an anchor (see Chapter 2, Anchoring). Fifty-fifty is a convenient heuristic, or mental shortcut, and people typically cannot adjust adequately, even once they can see that 50-50 was a completely inappropriate anchor to use.[30] Jonathan Baron gives the example of a person who says that since there is a risk of death from being trapped in a car by one's seatbelt, and there is also a risk of death in an accident that could have been prevented by the seatbelt, one should wear the seatbelt halfway on a long trip.[143] In this example of neglect of probability, two risks are treated as equivalent, even though the subject probably knows that the two outcomes are not of equal probability.

This effect is not confined to negative outcomes. People may rationalize that they have "a chance" of winning the lottery, and therefore it is worth playing.[141, 144] By failing to grasp how small the chance is, people may decide that the lottery is actually a good bet. As the theories of Sunstein and of Rottenstreich and Hsee suggest, the more vivid the mental image of the event, the greater the influence of a small chance of the event happening. Thus even if people do not overestimate the small probability, an emotionally arousing outcome is still likely to elicit greater sacrifices to avoid negative results or obtain positive results.

Salience (see Chapter 4) probably accounts for much of the inaccurate estimation of risk. Plane crashes and terrorism are well-covered in the media, precisely because they are very rare. Heart attacks and cancer are so common that they elicit much less sensational coverage. Thus the salience of rare events can be much higher, leading to overestimation of their probability.

Ironically, modern life may be falsely perceived as more risky than life in the past because we know of so many more possible risks. If each tiny risk is exaggerated, the sum of all the risks may seem to be huge, causing us to ignore the elimination or massive reduction in major diseases and causes of accident from the past. The smaller risks, such as radon exposure or fatal peanut allergies, may not have been known in past centuries, or would have seemed insignificant next to pandemic bubonic plague or smallpox.

Despite the general tendency to overestimate risks, sometimes people can decide to simply ignore a risk instead. Ignoring a risk is especially likely when taking a risk is inseparable from some benefit, so people who decide the benefit is worth the risk must learn to forget about the risk to avoid constantly suffering from anxiety (see Chapter 20, Ostrich effect). Adolescents are prone to ignore a wide variety of health risks to conform, to assert their independence, or for immediate gratification. Even adults are prone to ignore the health consequences of activities that are pleasurable. Strategies for dealing with risks ignored due to denial or mistrust of the medical system are presented in Chapter 20.

Applications in Medicine

Due to probability biases and patients' general tendency to be risk averse, it is difficult to describe risks of treatments with our patients in ways that put those risks in accurate perspective. Vague descriptions of uncommon risks are likely to be magnified out of proportion by most patients, leading to disproportionate fear of proposed treatment regimens. Precise language is needed that puts small risks into terms that a patient can understand. Emphasizing that a particular risk is similar to that of some familiar event may be a useful approach. Visual materials that communicate the true size of minuscule fractions can be very helpful as well.[12] Although poor adherence is always a concern, specific patterns of poor adherence may be caused by patients' overestimates of the risk of treatment. Resulting behaviors to avoid side effects may include using as little of the medication as possible and stopping the medication when partial improvement is observed.

If a patient shows a strong preference for not treating the disease at all to avoid risky drugs, we may want to emphasize that continuing to suffer with the disease is not a risk-free course of action either. Many disease processes already raise the risk of certain comorbidities greatly, while successful treatment of the disease greatly alleviates those risks. For example, patients with bipolar disorder are at high risk of dangerous behavior, such as drunk or reckless driving and other illegal acts. Psoriasis patients experience increased risk for obesity, metabolic syndrome, depression, and suicide. In these cases, successful treatment of the disease, even with treatments that are not risk-free, may actually reduce patients' overall risk of premature death.

We also need to be careful inadvertently confirming patients' misperceptions of treatment risk. Recently the authors had a patient in a clinical trial who believed that adalimumab was raising his blood sugar. If the patient found inaccurate information on the Internet and asked, "Do you think this drug might be what's causing my blood sugar to rise?" answering, "Yes, it might be" could reinforce the impression that the drug was a *likely* cause of the problem and make the patient resistant to any subsequent reassurance that adalimumab was not a likely cause of his rise in blood sugar. Answering the patient in a way that puts the probability in proper perspective may be prudent.

On the other hand, when patients request an unreasonably risky therapy — such as a biologic for mild arthritis that is not causing joint damage — giving the patient a more realistic understanding of the risk may be necessary. This may not require any more than reading the typical long list of side effects off the drug's package with a suitably alarmist tone of voice. We can also present relative risks; for example, "You have **ten times** as high a risk of heart attack with this drug!" may make a greater impact than explaining that the risk increases from 1/100,000 to 1/10,000. By skillfully using the right framing, we can tell patients there is a 999/1,000 chance of no adverse event when we want to reassure patients and 1/1,000 (or just, "there's a chance") of the same adverse event when we want to discourage them.

Quick Tips

- People tend to overemphasize rare risks, especially those that arouse strong emotion.
- Visual materials can help communicate the smallness of tiny risks.
- Presenting relative risks (e.g. "10 times as risky") often obscures the fact that absolute risks remain very low.

PART V

Willpower and its Depletion: How We Lose Control and Harm our Health

Chapter 22
Willpower and its Depletion
Scott A. Davis and Steven R. Feldman

One of the most maddening aspects of behavioral economics might be **depletion of our willpower**. Psychologists theorize that our willpower gradually gets depleted as more and more demands are made on it. A person who is tired from a long day at work is more likely to slip up and splurge on junk food than they would have been earlier in the day. Book chapters that appear toward the end of a book may get less attention than the first chapters, by both the editor and the reader. Depletion of willpower can cause people to have a lack of resources to make the healthy choice, but behavioral economics suggests some ways to limit the damage.

Background and History
The nature of willpower has fascinated psychologists for decades. A famous early discovery came from the Stanford marshmallow series of experiments, where psychologists gave young children a choice between eating one marshmallow now, or waiting 15 minutes and getting two marshmallows.[145, 146] Children's willpower, measured as their ability to defer gratification to get the two marshmallows, turned out to be highly predictive of future success.

Other experiments began to look at the effects of depleting willpower. For example, judges were more likely to make the default decision of not granting parole at times of day when they were depleted, while opting to grant parole at times when they were less depleted.[147] In an appalling failure of justice, the merits of the case affected the decision less than whether the judge had just had lunch.

Building on knowledge about willpower depletion, a team led by Roy Baumeister hypothesized that there was probably a biological mechanism for the depletion of willpower. Believing that depletion of blood glucose might be this mechanism, they did experiments in which subjects performed a task that depleted their willpower, then drank either a high-glucose drink or one sweetened with an artificial sweetener not containing glucose.[148] Subjects' performance on a subsequent task was better if they received the glucose drink, suggesting that blood glucose was an important part of the mechanism. Related experiments have demonstrated that people with depleted willpower are more likely to succumb to temptations of all kinds, including dishonesty.[21] Fortunately, willpower can be built up like a muscle, so that once a person becomes accustomed to resisting the temptation, failures become less and less common.[149]

Examples and Analysis

The implications of our behavior during times of depleted willpower are quite alarming. Politicians spend all day making important decisions that demand intense exertion of willpower. At the end of the day, they may have little willpower remaining to resist a bribe or sexual temptation. To help avoid unnecessary decisions that could deplete willpower, President Barack Obama wears only two colors of suits, avoiding having to make an extra decision each morning.[150]

Rational choice theory does not account for deficits of willpower. For example, traditional economic models suggest that we eat exactly the amount that we truly want, a quantity that is predetermined and not affected by whether or not we have recently been mentally taxed. Yet most of us actually are strongly influenced by how much food is in front of us and our level of willpower for resisting gluttony when deciding how much to eat. If the waiter brings more tortilla chips, we tend to eat them, unless we have the willpower to decline consumption or the wherewithal to decline the new basket of chips altogether.[151] When we don't have the willpower to control temptation, a smaller plate size may be helpful.[152]

Applications in Medicine

Patients struggle to make healthy decisions when depleted of willpower. Patients who are going through stressful life events often see worsening of chronic conditions they have had for years. While it could be that stress-induced effects on the immune system worsen patients' disease, it may be that the effects of stress on willpower to adhere to treatment plays a larger role in disease outcomes. Perhaps the best evidence of this is that when patients are hospitalized for treatment and adherence is assured, their condition may improve rapidly, even though their stress does not go away (despite our best efforts to make the hospital a comfortable, relaxing place).[56]

Direct Approaches: Strengthening Willpower

To minimize the effects of depletion, we need to make the medical visit as easy as possible for the patient. Offering comfortable chairs and a satisfying snack in the waiting room may not only improve patient satisfaction, but actually cause the patient to be more honest with us during the visit itself. If we must give the patient stressful tests during the visit, we might want to obtain vital information at the beginning of the visit, since the patient may be less honest after the tests. Overwhelming the patient with rapid-fire questions may also cause depletion, leading to less honest answers. Too much choice is depleting; when recommending treatments, offering a default option may reduce the psychological burden from having too much choice (see Chapter 6, Default option).

If we want to reduce overeating, having patients constantly resist temptation is not an ideal strategy. After making dozens of choices during a grocery shopping trip, many people are unable to resist the temptation to pick up some candy at the checkout aisle.[151] To avoid impulse purchases of unhealthy food, people can resolve to go to the grocery store only when they are not hungry, and avoid buffet restaurants with too many choices, since making numerous choices depletes willpower. Like the judges who make better decisions right after breakfast, people could also decide right after breakfast what they will have for dinner. Carving out one day a week where someone can indulge in otherwise forbidden foods is sometimes a way to give the willpower muscle some relaxation, as well as providing a sense of relief that they can look forward to. Thorgeirsson and Kawachi recommend three strategies specifically for dealing with bounded willpower: feedback (such as encouraging messages reinforcing the regimen), commitment contracts, and channel factors (e.g. showing people exactly how to perform the desired action, so they do not waste willpower deciding how to do it).[153] An example of channel factors is encouraging vaccination by giving students a campus map with the clinic clearly marked, so they do not get depleted by having to figure out where to go.[153] However, we have to be careful that patients are actually willing to perform the behavior, so that these strategies are not perceived as unwanted "shoves" rather than nudges.

For medication adherence, taking or applying medication at a quiet time of day, when willpower is not depleted, is likely to be the best approach. For a morning person, taking a medication first thing in the morning might be the easiest option, while other patients might feel less depleted if they waited until their morning coffee kicked in.

Indirect Approaches: Alternative Means to Address Problems of Low Willpower
When willpower is low, other strategies can be used to help encourage good health behaviors. To prevent overeating, we may want to suggest that patients put away their largest plates and serve food only on smaller plates. Alcoholic beverages can be served in tall, skinny glasses, which make a certain amount of alcohol look like more than it actually is.[154] The success of such nudges strongly influenced the campaign to limit portion sizes of sugary drinks in New York City to 16 ounces. This approach was consistent with libertarian paternalism, where people remain free to choose, but the choice architect paternalistically encourages the rational choice. Customers in New York City remained free to buy multiple drinks if they were very thirsty, but had to override the default of buying one 16-ounce drink; they were not automatically given a huge drink which they had to expend

willpower to avoid consuming. Recently, the ubiquitous "Nutrition Facts" labels on food items were revised to require the serving size to be expressed as the amount that the average cognitively-limited human would consume.[155] Thus, a label on a 20-ounce soda will now be based on the assumption that the consumer would show limited willpower and drink the whole thing, as most do. No longer will the average algebraically-challenged American have to solve a tricky, cognitively-depleting problem to figure out how many calories are in 1 pickle when the "serving size" is 3/4 pickle.

Like the size of plates, the size of prescriptions matters too. Patients given a larger prescription get a subconscious cue to use more, whereas with a smaller prescription, they would have to expend willpower to overcome their automatic tendency to use less. Patients obtain a greater proportion of 90-day prescriptions than the shorter 30-day prescriptions; mandating shorter prescriptions imposes a barrier to adherence.[156, 157] When patients are on multiple medications, syncing the time for them to be refilled will help minimize patient burden.

If we want patients to use a moisturizer liberally, we might want to suggest they go to a warehouse club like Costco and pick up a giant container of it. Seeing the large container every day sends the right message and prevents the patient from being reminded of the inconvenience of repeated trips to the store. However, we can also give a sample in our office so they can try it during the visit, preventing them from having to exert willpower to take the first dose. Moreover, sampling may prevent patients being unhappy that they bought a large container of something they didn't like.

Quick Tips

- People tend to slip into unhealthy behaviors after they have had to exert a great deal of willpower.

- Reducing stress on patients improves adherence and is likely to elicit more honest answers during a medical visit.

- To combat overeating, recommend serving food on smaller plates and beverages in tall, skinny glasses.

PART VI

Misperceptions of Time: How Past and Future Events Look Different

Chapter 23
Hyperbolic Discounting
Liz Ramsey, Scott A. Davis, and Steven R. Feldman

Every single day, each of us makes hundreds of thousands of decisions: the choice of waking up now to exercise or sleeping in, the choice to pay off our credit card fully or pay the minimum amount, the choice to wear sunscreen now or have a high risk of skin cancer later. These choices are far from meaningless; they can affect our health, our credit rating, our lifespan. Yet, many people may not choose what can objectively be seen as the better option in favor of the option that offers something now. Many of these "this now and that later" type decisions are based on "time discounting." Time discounting is the idea that many people give greater subjective value to a choice with immediate positive consequences compared to a choice with greater objective value but that involves waiting. The longer the wait, the more we discount the future benefit or risk; $100 today is worth more to us than a promise of $100 a year from now, which is in turn more valuable to us than a promise of $100 40 years from now.

Time discounting occurs in many common decisions. For example, your alarm clock goes off in the morning and you choose to hit snooze (immediate positive benefit) rather than jumping out of bed to hit the gym before work (greater but delayed benefit). Many of these decisions impact choices involved in health and healthcare; time discounting is combatted by every person currently on a diet, every smoker trying to quit, every uninsured patient deciding whether to pay to seek medical care. Overcoming the allure of an immediate benefit or avoiding an immediate cost is not easy, but is often the better choice overall. As physicians, by understanding tendencies to make time discounted decisions and incorporate strategies, we can help our patients overcome or manipulate these tendencies in their best interests.

Exponential versus hyperbolic discounting
Standard economic theory uses exponential discounting to provide a mathematical foundation for understanding time delayed choice behaviors. In these models, people have consistent choices over time. If someone prefers X now over Y a month from now, they would also prefer X 12 months from now over Y 13 months from now.[a]

Many times, human choices do not correspond to this model of behavior. Consider the following example. If a person is offered the choice between being given $100 today or $150 one month from today, many will choose the $100. But if the same person were offered $100 one year from today or $150 13

---

[a] In such models the current value $V_X(0)$ of some future state $V_X(t)$, where X is a given amount of money, would be estimated as the future value at time t, $V_X(t)$, multiplied by $e^{-\sigma t}$ where σ is the discount rate: $V_X(0)=V_X(t)e^{-\sigma t}$. This mathematical formulation of discounting leads to consistent choices over time. If someone prefers $X in the future (time t) over $Y now, [mathematically expressed as $V_X(t)>V_Y(0)$] then they would make the same choice if the same options were presented at some other time t′ later [mathematically expressed as $V_X(t+t')> V_Y(t')$]. This is true because $V_X(t+t')= V_X(t)e^{-\sigma t+t'}= V_X(t)e^{-\sigma t}e^{-\sigma t'}$ and $V_Y(t')= V_Y(0)e^{-\sigma t'}$. Since $e^{-\sigma t'}$ is a constant, then $V_X(t)> V_Y(0)$ implies that $V_X(t)e^{-\sigma t'}> V_Y(0)e^{-\sigma t'}$.

months from today they would likely choose the $150. Both the reward amounts and the time difference between receiving those amounts are equal to the first example ($50 more with an extra 30 days of wait). However, in this second scenario, people often choose to wait for the later reward. Why? What has changed from the first scenario? The difference between the two scenarios is that the person now views both rewards as distant; in the first example, only the later reward was perceived to be distant. This scenario is an example of hyperbolic discounting. Hyperbolic discounting postulates that people place high value on immediately available events; people will wait for the superior option if they do not perceive either option to be occurring immediately. David Laibson writes, "Hyperbolic discount functions are characterized by a relatively high discount rate over short horizons and a relatively low discount rate over long horizons" [158]. A high discount rate correlates to a choice for the inferior but immediate option — because the superior option's value is discounted because of the need to wait for it.

Background and History

The concept of hyperbolic discounting was developed to explain "impulsiveness." People prefer to have benefits now rather than wait for them in the future. Originally, this phenomenon was thought to be well-explained using an exponential mathematical function:

$$\text{Value} = \text{Amount} \times (1 - \text{Rate})^{\text{Delay}}$$

However, this model did not explain how dramatically future values are discounted. If an exponential model accurately described time discounting, then there would never be a change in preference to an inferior reward, even if it were immediately available (Figure 1A); the value of the larger reward would always be greater.

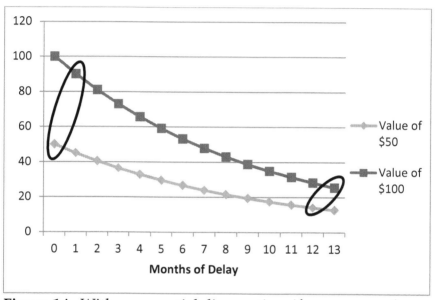

Figure 1A. With exponential discounting, if a person prefers something now over something else a month from now, they would also make the same choice 12 months vs 13 months from now. With a constant 10% per month discounting rate, the larger prize *n+1* months later is always worth 80% more than the smaller prize at *n* months.

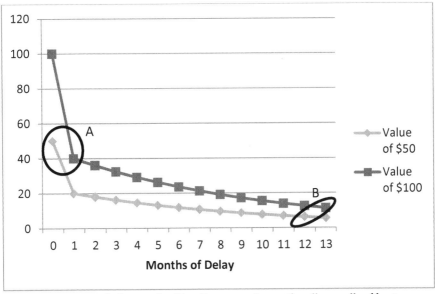

Figure 1B. With hyperbolic discounting, the "now" effect makes the smaller prize <u>now</u> worth more than the larger prize at 1 month delay (circle A). The value of the larger prize plummets disproportionately in the first month of delay, making it less desirable than a smaller prize <u>now</u>. However, since the difference between a delay of 12 months and 13 months is not as psychologically important, the smaller prize at 12 months delay is still worth less than the larger prize at 13 months (circle B).

In contrast, if a hyperbolic function
$$Value=Amount/(1+K \times Delay)$$
were the correct model, there could be changes in preference
over time that would make people prefer an immediate
inferior reward (Figure 1B). The hyperbolic function shows
that at time t=0 when both rewards are distant, the larger
reward is preferred. However, as time (t) approaches the
smaller reward, it becomes preferred — this reward is viewed
by the participant as immediate in comparison to the larger
reward. After the time at which the small reward is given, the
larger reward is once again preferred.

Ainslie postulated that only a hyperbolic curve, not an
exponential one, was concave enough to accurately represent
human nature of time discounting. Ainslie examined research
in the fields of economics [159], sociology [160], analytical
psychiatry [161, 162], behavioral psychology [163], and behavior
therapy [164, 165], all of which suggested a curve more concave
than an exponential function to illustrate time discounting.
Ideas from all of these fields suggested that a hyperbolic curve
was the only way to explain the time-inconsistent choices
made by both humans and animals in the experiments of
various fields.

Examples and Analysis
Examples of time discounting are ubiquitous in modern
culture, medicine included. Discounting can explain the desire
of people to pay for a large purchase on a monthly basis —
even if they have to pay a higher total cumulative amount —
than to buy something less expensive that they could afford
outright. The positive immediate effect of paying nothing for

the product initially dominates over the more distant but more positive effect of a lower total price paid. The United States government has implemented policies to protect its citizens from their own hyperbolic discounting. Left to their own devices, the majority of Americans would spend now instead of saving for later, leaving them destitute after retirement or if a serious injury were to render us unable to work. Instead, the government forces us to save money now, via the social security system and Medicare.[166] Hyperbolic discounting explains these examples: workers must choose between spending money now (lesser but immediate reward) and saving for later (larger but distant benefit). When the lesser option is immediate and the greater option is distant, the inferior choice will be made. Without these imposed systems, most people would continue to make the inferior, immediate choice month after month and would therefore never accumulate enough savings to support themselves when they are retired or disabled.

Applications in Medicine

Many more examples of time discounting can be found throughout the medical field. Teenagers usually have a high rate of discounting; they often choose to sunbathe all summer to receive the immediate effect of a desirable tan instead of the greater, but distant positive effect of skin health. Type 2 diabetics, who despite adequate education and resources, do not make major lifestyle changes are choosing the short-term effect of tasty foods and avoiding exercising over the longer-term positive effects of a healthier life and fewer complications. One of the biggest applications of time discounting in medicine is the example of alcohol, cigarette, or drug addicts. Many addicts fall victim to discounting and choose the immediate effect of the high or buzz over a long-term benefit of health and happiness. However, if the choice were instead between using the drug of choice one year from now and being sober one year from now, recovering addicts would be expected to choose the second option. In this way, hyperbolic discounting "sets up a conflict between today's preferences, and the preferences that will be held in the future" [158]. Compared to controls, heavy social drinkers [167], smokers [168, 169], opioid users [170, 171], and methamphetamine-dependent individuals [172] are said to display "steep discounting". Steep discounting describes an individual for whom time to wait is a much more important factor in decision-making than it may be in others. These people assess large value discounts to any option that is not immediate. Although causality has not been established from these studies, they do show a correlation of personality types with steep discounting tendencies and the substance abuse.

Clearly, time discounting leads to many choices that are not in the patient's best interest in the long-term. In addition, physicians often have difficulty understanding and empathizing with patients who make choices according to this model. Physicians, who spend more than a decade in training, tend to excel in "delayed gratification" situations. It might be said that we have very shallow discounting styles since we are apparently very willing to wait for a great reward. Therefore, it may be difficult for us to understand the preference of many of our patients for the inferior, immediate choice. How then, can we not only understand but also manipulate principles of time discounting to our patients' advantage? We must first accept that patients will often operate by basic time-discounting principles. If we can accept this fact, much frustration can be avoided. Additionally, we can use time discounting principles to re-frame the narrative of lifestyle choices. For example, when prescribing anti-depressants, it may be beneficial to identify for the patient an immediate reward, like the sense of entitlement and self-reliance that the patient will feel upon taking control of his health. Framing this idea of empowerment as the positive, immediate consequence of taking the medication will help the patient to make this choice. Otherwise, the patient may set his own narrative: that a positive, immediate reward of saving money can be found in not taking the medication.

An established method of combatting time discounting in addicts involves forming "bundles" or "sets" [172]. It is based on Aristotle's idea that choosing the immediate-small reward was the result of choosing based on "particulars" instead of "universals" [173]. By this token, less impulsive decisions will be made if one considers the decision as part of a universal truth or choice rather than considering it as one single decision. For addicts, instructing them to conceptualize each decision to avoid or use the drug of choice as part of a set of decisions may decrease usage. Addicts tend to consider each decision to use their drug again as an exception — "I'll just use today since it's been a tough day" or "If I just use one more time, I'll be ready to quit for good." Training people to view each temptation to use their drug as a challenge to their general principle of "I use drugs" or "I do not use drugs" will decrease impulsive behavior [174]. Such strategies can also be employed in medication or treatment adherence. Having the patient identify themselves as either compliant with their doctor's advice or noncompliant may help them see the daily task of taking medicines as part of a "universal rule."

Quick Tips

- Future payoffs are perceived as less valuable, causing people to prefer smaller rewards that are immediate.
- Emphasizing immediate rewards of a regimen may help patients who would not be willing to wait for a long-term reward.
- Conceptualizing a decision as part of a general principle (being a person who performs healthy behavior) can help overcome impulsive behavior.

Chapter 24
Rosy Retrospection
Noah Z. Feldman

Rosy Retrospection is the tendency to misremember past events more positively than they actually were. The most common example is that of family trips. During the excursion small annoyances, frustrations, and anxieties abound: forgetting where the car keys are, scraping a knee, losing the sunglasses, etc. This drives a negative experience *in the moment*. While such annoyances are common, when the trip is remembered after many years the minor annoyances will be forgotten in favor of the positive things that stand out: a panoramic view, watching the geysers, seeing a moose, etc. These experiences power a much more positive memory of the trip. This is why you could hate the trip you went on when you were a kid yet still drag your own progeny on the same less than joyous journey.

Background and History
The idea of Rosy Retrospection has existed for a long time, but it was first studied by Mitchell, Thompson, Cronk, and Peterson.[175] They surveyed participants about a trip before they left, while they were there, and after they returned; the questions they asked included what they specifically planned on, were experiencing, or remembered, as well as their general perception of the vacation. They included three separate experiments: a tour of Europe, Thanksgiving break, and a three-week trans-Californian bike ride. They found that people had high hopes for upcoming trips, valuing them

highly before leaving, as well as positive memories afterwards, for example feeling, "I remember all the fun we had on our little excursion"; Participants however were largely negative about their vacations while they were in the midst of them, citing annoyances and frustrations that were lessening the experience.

There are a number of explanations for why people are biased in this way.[176] The first (and most common) is that while people may suffer annoyances in the moment, they forget those annoyances and later remember that it was "a wholly enjoyable experience." Another is that when vacationers look forward to wonderful trips where nothing unexpected happens and eventually things do go wrong, they remember not only the less than sublime trip, but also the heavenly experience that they expected to have. One last explanation, that of "Dissonance," predicts that people were expecting an experience much better than what they received, so, to protect themselves from the idea that their judgment was faulty, they misremember the actual events as closer to their predictions.

Examples and Analysis
Rosy Retrospection is not limited to minor annoyances. Many advanced mountain climbers describe their experiences during the climb as "… harshly uncomfortable, miserable, and exhausting…", but when they reach the top, the memories of pride and joy override any of hardship. One important caveat in Rosy Retrospection is that it can work the other way. When expecting things to be negative, minor positive aspects may be forgotten; this makes you misremember bad situations as worse than they actually were, the opposite of Rosy

Retrospection.

Many things can invoke this effect. A trip to the theater involving a bumper crop of annoyances from traffic to overpriced popcorn will often be forgotten when juxtaposed with a few awesome moments enjoyed on screen. When asked at any point if they were enjoying their trip, most moviegoers give a lukewarm impression, but, when asked at the a day later about the experience in general, they will give a rating that is often better than **any** that they gave during the film.[176] The real measure for when Rosy Retrospection can or cannot be seen lies in simple test: If a person actively seeks out an experience where the benefits are felt during the experience, they will misremember the situation as better than it actually was.

Rosy Retrospection falls into a larger class of biases related to how the mind interprets series of events that occur over time. People do not simply add up the sum total of all the joys and pains in an experience to come up with their overall assessment of a series of events.[177] Global retrospective evaluations are heavily influenced by peak experiences and by final experiences. For example, in a study of colonoscopy, patients' overall report of the pain associated with the procedure was predicted by the average of the most intense pain and the pain over the final 3 minutes of the procedure. Patients also prefer trends toward improvement; pain that goes from 3-2-1 is preferred over pain going from 1-2-3, even though the absolute amount of pain is the same in both cases. Perhaps surprisingly, patients tend to retrospectively report less discomfort in a sequence of pain like {2, 5, 8, 4} over {2, 5,

8}, even though mathematically there is clearly less absolute pain experienced in the latter sequence than in the former. When performing painful procedures, patients' memories of the experience will be better if the most painful portion of the procedure occurs early, rather than late, in the process.

Table 1. Situations in which Rosy Retrospection is more or less likely to occur

More likely
• There are many small annoyances or negative surprises within the experience
• The experience was positively anticipated for a long time
• More time has passed since the experience
• The peak and the end of the experience are very positive
Less likely
• Expectations were low before the experience
• The experience was joined involuntarily
• With ongoing processes as opposed to singular events

Applications in Medicine
Rosy Retrospection has a number of potential effects in medical care. One such effect is that patients will gradually forget small annoyances in taking the medications that they used before if there had been some more significant benefit; they may begin to become nostalgic for and want to return to the previous medicine that they had previously quit. We can help to avert this by reminding the patient of difficulties of the old medications, bringing those minor annoyances back to the forefront. Patients might also slowly devalue the pains of a

minor ailment that has been in remission for a long time; part of our role is to keep them aware of this as a means to encourage better adherence to treatment.

There is another significant effect of rosy retrospection. Imagine you are a patient anticipating a positive experience with a new specialist, but find that there are endless minor hassles to make an appointment: You are unable to find a parking spot, the magazines in the waiting room were beyond out of date, and the examination room was absolutely frosty (and you are dressed in only a very lightweight examination gown). Your new doctor comes in and delivers the best possible one-on-one, personal experience. He or she is friendly and engaged, looks at all your symptoms knowledgeably, and builds a beautifully clear tapestry out of your treatment options. You then face a problem with paying at the check out desk, dodge around a massive spill of (what you hope is) water, and get stuck in traffic on your way out. A few weeks later when a friend asks if you would suggest that same physician, you would probably, without pause, give a resounding yes. Rosy Retrospection has caused you to devalue the small annoyances, leaving you with a positive view driven by the great one-on-one experience. This effect means that a doctor who can create a truly perfect connection for the few minutes he or she has with his or her patients can overcome obstacles like poor funding and overworked staff. Still, knowing that patients place emphasis on final events, it may be best to have the most personable of those staff members working at the check out desk rather than the check in desk.

Quick Tips

- Past experiences are viewed more positively than they were viewed at the time, especially if they have a great peak experience and ending.
- To maximize patient satisfaction, avoid having the most painful event occur near the end of the visit.
- Patients tend to forget minor annoyances, which may cause them view a previous medication more favorably than the current one.

Chapter 25
Regret
Scott A. Davis

Regret is a negative feeling occurring when people look back
on past actions. Although it has the positive function of
causing people to consider how they might avoid repeating
prior mistakes, regret can also be a very powerful factor
motivating people to perform irrational actions. Regret leads
people to compare a situation to an alternative that they
imagine would have resulted if they had made a different
decision. As with the situation where comparing ourselves to
others makes us depressed (see Chapter 18, Hedonic
treadmill), comparing our situation to a counterfactual can
lead to a great deal of regret, which we sometimes even
anticipate and try to avoid. Fortunately, at times anticipated
regret can actually be exploited to improve patients'
participation in beneficial health behaviors.

Background and History
Historically, regret was generally assumed to be a strictly
negative emotion that was equally unpleasant compared to
other negative emotions. Recent psychological literature has
challenged this assumption and shown that regret has key
positive functions which people value, such as motivating
people to avoid repeating their mistakes in the future.[178] In a
2008 study, participants rated regret as the most positive of
eight negative emotions.[178] They also rated it as the best
emotion to accomplish the functions of "placing past events in
context, preparing to engage in approach and in avoidance

behaviors, gaining insight into one's own past behavior and current disposition, and also in facilitating smoother social relations."[178] In short, people value regret for helping them learn from their mistakes, especially when they have accidentally hurt others.

People can even anticipate future regret and modify current behavior as a result. In fact, they often tend to overestimate future regret, an effect labeled by Daniel Gilbert and colleagues as "buying emotional insurance that they do not actually need."[179] The "emotional insurance" may even be literal insurance with a real monetary cost, such as an extended warranty on a car. In reality, Gilbert and colleagues showed that people usually do not blame themselves as much as they originally expected for the eventual outcome, blaming some other person or cause instead, or rationalizing that the outcome was not as bad as originally thought.[179] For example, if a student gets into the University of Chicago but is rejected from Harvard, she might start to view Chicago more positively and Harvard more negatively, persuading herself retrospectively that she would have chosen Chicago even if she had been admitted to both schools.

Examples and Analysis

Despite the extensive psychological study of regret, analysis of it from a behavioral economics standpoint is comparatively recent. Dan Ariely writes that regret is something of a unique feeling since "it means that your happiness is not influenced by your actual state, but by the ease of imagining a state that you are not in."[180] The ease of imagining differs based on how different the actual event was from the counterfactual:

Imagine, for example, that you missed your flight either by two minutes, or by two hours: under which of these conditions would you be more upset? Most likely, you will feel more upset if you missed your flight by two minutes. Why? After all, your actual state is the same: in both cases you are stuck at Newark for five hours waiting for the next flight, watching the same news report on CNN, responding to email on your smartphone, and munching on expensive and not very good food. They key is that having missed your flight by just a few minutes, you continuously think about all the things you might have done to get on the plane on time – leaving the house five minutes earlier, checking your route to avoid traffic jams, and so on. This comparison to how things could have been, and the feeling of "almost" makes you miserable. By contrast, a two-hour delay is not as upsetting because you don't make these kinds of regretful, "woulda, coulda, shoulda" comparisons.[181]

Another example is that a person who does not normally play the lottery could be induced to participate when a friend has already bought tickets and offers to sell some. Thinking about how regretful they would feel if they turned down the offer and their friend won, the person is likely to buy the ticket.[182]

Applications in Medicine

Although regret can have very negative psychological consequences for some patients, anticipated regret can actually have benefits that we can use. Some public health agencies actually try to take advantage of people's tendency toward anticipated regret to increase screening rates for certain cancers.[183] By merely giving a questionnaire that included questions on whether the patient would feel regret if they did not participate in the screening, the rate of participation in cervical cancer screenings in one region of England increased from 44% to 65%.[183] The same intervention improved organ donation rates in a subsequent study.[184] Family members are less likely to veto their deceased relative's decision to donate organs when asked questions that invoke anticipated regret.[185] Perhaps to improve adherence, hypertensive patients could be asked in similar fashion, "How would you feel if you didn't take your medication and then had a heart attack?"

If a patient is very reluctant to try an effective treatment, we could ask how they would feel if they continued to suffer from their condition when an effective treatment was available to them. We could elicit their favorite outdoor activities and then ask, for example, "Would you feel regret if you weren't able to enjoy hiking this year because we didn't get your COPD under control?" Similar to the lottery example where friends had already bought tickets, we could say to a patient who enjoys travel, "Would it be disappointing if you weren't able to participate in that once-in-a-lifetime river cruise down the Yangtze with your friends?"

As Ariely's missed flight example predicts, people are more likely to be influenced by regret when the counterfactual is easy to imagine, such as when the flight was missed by two minutes. If a patient is taking many of the steps necessary to improve health but not others, we should therefore emphasize how they are "almost" fully successful, making it easier to visualize the needed change. For example, if an obese patient who had bariatric surgery has already changed their diet tremendously and started exercising, but is struggling to take their post-operative vitamins correctly, we should emphasize all the things they have done right, and thus how small a step they still need to take. We could say something like, "Now that you have done so much to look so great, would you regret if you got vitamin deficiency and weren't able to enjoy your health to the fullest? Let's develop a plan to help you remember to take the vitamins."

Sometimes a patient will tend to ignore the overall success and be fixated on one failure, such as the Olympic silver medalist who devalues the accomplishment and wallows in regret about not having won the gold.[186] A cosmetic dental patient who started with severe fluorosis might ignore a 90% reduction in tooth discoloration and obsess over the tiny amount of yellow coloration that cannot be eliminated. Identifying patients with unrealistic expectations before performing cosmetic procedures, and turning them down if their expectation of unreasonable results cannot be changed, might be the best strategy for preventing this type of irrational post-procedural regret.[187]

Although regret sometimes serves a positive function, we must also remember that patients and their caregivers can be devastated by feelings of regret. An excellent example is a situation where a patient with a heart condition arrives in the ER and dies almost immediately*. The caregiver asks, "Would it have made a difference if I had brought him in yesterday?"

If we give any answer other than "No, it wouldn't have made any difference," we risk sentencing the caregiver to a lifetime of regret for not bringing the patient in sooner. This is a case where we need to safeguard someone's feelings, even at the risk of not telling the full story. Even if we said there was only a small chance it would have helped, the caregiver would likely obsess over that small chance and feel responsible for the patient's death.

Regret is frequently associated with saying, "I'm sorry." Some of us may be inclined to interpret this statement as admission of fault and not want to say it, but it can be said as a strong expression of empathy without taking responsibility for the bad outcome. If there is any ambiguity, we can say something like, "I'm sorry you had this outcome," while making clear that we followed normal procedure and cannot prevent every bad outcome. This simple statement of regret restores the feeling that the patient saw a friendly, caring doctor – the leading predictor of whether patients were satisfied in the DrScore.com patient survey.[47]

Quick Tips

> - People value the emotion of regret for helping them avoid repeating past mistakes.
> - Asking patients about whether they would feel regret can help improve participation in healthy behaviors, such as cancer screening.
> - Expressing regret for a bad outcome is a powerful statement of caring, even when we could not have prevented the bad outcome.

*The authors are indebted to Ralph "Monty" Leonard, PhD, MD, for this example.

Chapter 26
Procrastination
Noah Z. Feldman

To write this book, the lead authors divided up its chapters between a number of associates, each assigned to complete their section and then send them back to be edited and formatted. We made the list of concepts in early November, to be sent in by February. This open schedule was decided upon because it would reduce the stress on the editors by letting them go over the articles one at a time as they rolled in instead of in one huge block at the end. As of this writing however, the New Year has rolled around and few of the chapters had been completed and sent in to the editors. This unfortunate state of affairs reminded us of one last chapter to include on an important aspect of human behavior— procrastination— a behavior that can sabotage patient treatment outcomes, as well as our book publishing goals.

Procrastination occurs when people delay the completion of a task even when they gain nothing from the delay (that is, when standard economic models would predict that they wouldn't delay). Whether working on an art project, trying to floss our teeth, or even writing a chapter for a book of applied behavioral economics, humans have a tendency to put off work.

Background and History
Depending on your perspective, procrastination is either as old as the first hunter who decided that "this spear will last

one more turn of the moon", or as ancient as the prehistoric fish who thought to himself, I'm going to try out this whole "land" thing tomorrow. A little closer to home, a prototypic study of procrastination was done by a college professor trying to improve his student's essays.[188] Each student was asked to do three essays by the end of the semester, each of which was short and generally quite easy. Every year, the students came with pencils sharpened and notebooks open, firmly believing that they would not procrastinate, that they would write their essays on time and give them the full attention they deserved. However, every single year they would fall behind and many would turn in all three essays on the last day, having printed them that morning. To improve grades (and reduce the number of essays he had to grade at once), the professor split the students into three groups. The first group (the control) was under the old system, turning in their papers at any time before the end of the course. The second group had deadlines for their papers evenly distributed throughout the year (at one third intervals, one essay falling at the very end); turning essays in after these deadlines would incur a small daily penalty. The third group was told that they could chose whatever turn-in deadline dates they wanted, but that those dates would be publicly declared, unmovable, and subject to the same penalties for tardiness.

Considering that there is no penalty for turning papers in early, standard economic theory dictates that students in the third group should choose their turn-in due dates at the end of the semester, giving themselves the most flexibility. However, the vast majority (88%) did not do so, generally placing their due dates about one week after those of the second group. Thus, students predicted their own tendencies to procrastinate and set their schedules accordingly.

The results of this experiment were rather staggering. As predicted, the second group— the group with predefined, evenly spaced, intermediate deadlines— did slightly better than the control group; the intermediate deadline group still procrastinated some, starting even a little bit closer to the deadline for each essay; this made sense considering that it's easier to do three last minute tasks separately than to do them at the same time. The improvements for the third group were much more significant however. They would often turn in their essays *before* the due date they set for themselves, often by as much as a week, and the quality of their essays was markedly higher, as they did not rush their work. Several factors may explain why students in the third group had the best essay timing results: first, students in the third group understood their own schedules and would set their due dates after they would have a block of time that had a lower workload; second, this third group had their decisions publicly announced, so everyone would know if they failed, creating a social pressure to succeed; third, students had set the due date themselves, so they could not argue that they "hadn't been given enough time" or that "the professor was unfair with the scheduling": finally, by starting the essay writing process with the deadline setting procedure, the professor imbued the whole semester with a sense of agency. The students felt that they succeeded or failed by their own efforts, making them emotionally invested in their success.

Examples and Analysis

Procrastinating on health related actions is a problem. To understand this problem better, and potential solutions, we can look at procrastinating on financial issues, in particular, procrastinating on saving for retirement. In many jobs, workers often neglect paying into sorely needed savings, procrastinating retirement saving. They fail to build a safety net and often live just above the poverty line after their employment ends. Underfunding for retirement is an important problem that has been studied and can provide insights into factors that underlie procrastination. Four basic causes of procrastination on retirement savings have been identified: hyperbolic discounting, bounded rationality, inertia, and nominal loss aversion.

The first factor, hyperbolic discounting (discussed in detail in Chapter 23), is a rather unintuitive but powerful facet of human decision making, that humans value current events very much greater than future events. An early human might have preferred to build his house tomorrow rather than today, because he might be dead by tomorrow. Hyperbolic discounting is best exemplified by noting that if someone were given the choice to get $100 one year from now or $120 one month later, they would likely say they would prefer the $120; however if given the choice between $100 now and $120 a month from now, they would take the $100. People can see that it is better to wait one more month for the extra $20 as long as it is far in the future, but getting the $100 now is too good to pass up. Today, given the choice between spending and having fun today versus spending and having fun in the future, people undervalue future spending and don't save now to pay for future spending.

Bounded rationality is the idea that people do not have infinite computational power at their disposal, and thus cannot adequately judge the variety of future options; in situations too complicated to find the rational solution, the mind switches to gut reactions, which is (among other things) influenced even more by hyperbolic discounting and inertia. Calculations of funding future retirement is complicated, leading to procrastination. Inertia causes people in a particular state to stay in that state; change requires mental effort, and it is easier to just procrastinate and not start a new savings program (inertia can be put to good use if participating in a retirement program is the default option, as discussed in Chapter 6). Finally, there is loss aversion (discussed in Chapter 13); people dislike lowering their current income. The feeling of loss of current spending ability causes people to procrastinate and put off saving for the future for the future.

Researchers sought to design a system to fight this financial procrastination and found an effective way to encourage retirement plan participation.[189] In so doing they provide a great example of how to reduce procrastination. Combining ideas about the causes of procrastination, the researchers designed a system called the Save More Tomorrow Plan (SMT) in which the employees would have an optimal amount (the amount the corporations standing savings policy would match, and no greater than the pay increase) of each successive raise saved automatically, removed directly from their paycheck; significantly, every worker who took part in this plan had previously disagreed with a plan that would have them accept a 5% pay cut. The pre-specified increases in retirement savings were designed to specifically mitigate the effects of bounded rationality, because workers were not expected to do any of the math themselves, and the automatic nature of the increase helped to reduce inertia. The aversion to losses was combatted by having increases in retirement savings occur at the time of pay raises, so that the amount of monthly take home pay never dropped. Perhaps most importantly, the plan dealt with hyperbolic discounting by having workers make the decision to participate almost three months before the first subtraction would take place.

This approach was monumentally effective. The majority of workers (roughly 80%) stayed with the program to its completion, at which point they were putting away about 12% of their income, the highest their company would match, far higher than any of their peers, and much more than they had previously said was their maximum. Even those that did drop out did not lower their savings rate back to its original level, so those that dropped out in the second year still benefitted. To boil it down to its simplest, the plan has people **pre-commit** to **immediately** use any **unexpected boon** on a task you might otherwise procrastinate on: make a pact with yourself that if you get a snow day you will use it to work on cleaning up the house (or finishing this chapter), preplan to write up your research while waiting at a restaurant, put in place a plan that forces yourself to save any money you get from a raffle you entered.

One of the reasons that procrastination is so prevalent is the fact that the way we value different actions fluctuates with what action we are doing, **in that moment.** We value sexual release more when we are sexually charged.[190] We think Facebook is more valuable, the social connections seem more meaningful, when we actually look at that white and blue page. Thus, when we are thinking about how little we get done, computer games and other diversions seem like complete wastes of time, while in the moment they feel like a well-deserved break or a necessary return to the world. Or seen from the mind from a person who is currently procrastinating, abstinence from those diversionary activities feels both ludicrous and implausible. Don't take this as a statement in support of procrastination, but as an impetus to engage in thought over why you would procrastinate, as a person must know his enemy if it is to be defeated (by the way, too much internal thought can also be a potent form of procrastination).

Applications in Medicine
Approaches used to circumvent procrastinating on important financial actions can also be used to reduce procrastination on important medical actions (and to get people to finish writing their book chapters). We observed several steps that can be generalized:

- Pre-commit to start the plan in the future, because people may not be willing to commit to start the plan now if it interferes with the things they want to do now.
- As much as possible, avoid framing the activities in the plan as losses

- Make as much of the process automatic as possible so that people don't have to make an active choice for the desired event or behavior to occur.

As for writing research papers and book articles, our own process would probably serve as an excellent guideline. After realizing that production of book chapters was too slow for the book to be completed in a timely way, the editors decided to employ a staggered workload system. They created a Google docs page with each of the articles to be written, with the name of the writer next to it; they then attached the date that the worker said each stage would be finished. Thus, they efficiently established a series of achievable goals, public announcement of the goals, and responsibility for their completion. After this system was put in place, the chapters started rolling in, many arriving even before the predicted completion date, and before long there was time left for an extra chapter on the very subject of procrastination. Another anti-procrastination strategy we employed, which has helped with getting the book completed, was to ask authors to turn in an outline within 1 week of signing up. This may indicate that getting people to start an action is hugely important. Once they have completed a small part of a task, loss aversion may kick in: if they abandoned the project after having put some effort into it, they would likely feel they had wasted the time that they spent on this first step. In addition, we were able to tell within the first 1 week whether an author's usual practice was to procrastinate or to do things on time.

Patients will often delay taking their medicines. They decide it takes too long for them to put ointments on in the morning, but the afternoon would be perfect; then in the afternoon they decide that they would rub off while they sleep so they should wait for the morning. By having patients verbally commit to take the medications at a specific time -"I will take it at 8:00 every morning"- you can help to evade this procrastinatory spiral; were there a machine to automatically apply the product, all the better. Sometimes a friend or family member can fulfill this role.

Patients may procrastinate and put off medical examinations. Setting up a return appointment or a procedure like colonoscopy one year in the future is easier for patients to commit to (because it is in the future) and much more likely to result in a visit than to expect patients to go to the effort a year from now to schedule an appointment or procedure when they need it.

Procrastination takes effect in numerous everyday struggles. Consider exercise regimens and dietary changes. Common thoughts like "one more slice of cheesecake won't ruin my life" or " I can start exercising tomorrow" are great measurements of when procrastination is getting ahead of you. An individual indulgence seems to have no effect long-term because it is so minimal; but the effect is major when you consider that this is a pattern of behavior affecting the rest of your life. Other strategies discussed in this chapter may help. Pre-commit to small steps of progress on a series of intervals. Commit publicly and create accountability to meeting commitments. Make the changes automatic (stay away from places that have cheesecake on the menu).

Reference List

(1) Kahneman D, Tversky A. Choices, Values, and Frames. *Am Psychologist* 1984;39(4):341-350.

(2) Investopedia. Anchoring. *http://www.investopedia.com/terms/a/anchoring.asp.* 2009 December 1. Accessed December 7, 2013.

(3) Tversky A, Kahneman D. Judgment under Uncertainty: Heuristics and Biases. *Science* 1974;185(4157):1124-1131.

(4) Ariely D. *Predictably Irrational: The Hidden Forces that Shape Our Decisions.* New York: HarperCollins; 2008.

(5) Kahneman D. *Thinking, Fast and Slow.* New York: Farrar, Straus and Giroux; 2013.

(6) Pynchon V. The power of framing and anchors. *http://www.negotiationlawblog.com/negotiation/the-power-of-framing-and-anchors/.* 2007 June 25. Accessed December 7, 2013.

(7) Ariely D. This is how I feel about buying apps. *http://danariely.com/2011/12/25/the-oatmeal-this-is-how-i-feel-about-buying-apps/.* 2011 December 25. Accessed December 7, 2013.

(8) Clifford S, Rampell C. Sometimes we want prices to fool us. *http://www.nytimes.com/2013/04/14/business/for-penney-a-tough-lesson-in-shopper-psychology.html.* 2013 April 13. Accessed December 7, 2013.

(9) Nudge blog. How one call center uses anchoring in its customer service. *http://nudges.org/2010/08/05/how-one-call-center-uses-anchoring-in-its-customer-service/*. 2010 August 5. Accessed December 7, 2013.

(10) Hartzband P, Groopman J. Three major cognitive errors physicians make. *http://www.kevinmd.com/blog/2011/10/major-cognitive-errors-physicians.html*. 2011 October 9. Accessed December 7, 2013.

(11) Astion M. Medical errors and the way doctors think. *http://www.aacc.org/publications/cln/2009/october/Pages/1009_safety5.aspx*. 2009 October 11. Accessed December 7, 2013.

(12) Kaminska E, Patel I, Dabade TS et al. Comparing the lifetime risks of TNF-alpha inhibitor use to common benchmarks of risk. *J Dermatolog Treat* 2013;24(2):101-106.

(13) WebMD. Sclerotherapy for Varicose and Spider Veins. *http://www.webmd.com/skin-problems-and-treatments/sclerotherapy-for-varicose-veins*. 2012 July 11. Accessed December 7, 2013.

(14) Schlessinger J. Navigating the pricing pressures of cosmetic injectables. *Practical Dermatology* 2013;10(10):22-24.

(15) Verbitsky AA, Kalashnikov VG. Category of Context and Contextual Approach in Psychology. *Psychol Russia State of the Art* 2012;117-129.

(16) Hechter M, Kanazawa S. Sociological Rational Choice Theory. *Annu Rev Sociol* 1997;23:191-214.

(17) Green SL. Rational Choice Theory: An Overview. 2002; 2002.

(18) Rysiew P. Relativism and Contextualism. In: Hales SD, editor. *A Companion to Relativism*. Blackwell; 2011. 286-305.

(19) Ariely D, Loewenstein GF, Prelec D. Tom Sawyer and the construction of value. *J Econ Behav Org* 2006;60:1-10.

(20) Kienle A, Lilge L, Vitkin AI. Why do veins appear blue? A new look at an old question. *Appl Optics* 1996;35(7):1151-1160.

(21) Ariely D. *The (Honest) Truth About Dishonesty: How We Lie to Everyone -- Especially Ourselves*. New York: HarperCollins; 2012.

(22) Duhigg C. *The Power of Habit*. New York: Random House; 2012.

(23) Hamilton R, Chernev A. The Impact of Product Line Extensions and Consumer Mindset on the Formation of Price Image. *J Market Res* 2010;47(1):51-62.

(24) Mills EJ, Nachega JB, Buchan I et al. Adherence to antiretroviral therapy in sub-Saharan Africa and North America: a meta-analysis. *JAMA* 2006;296(6):679-690.

(25) Shiffrin RM, Schneider W. Controlled and Automatic Human Information Processing: II. Perceptual Learning, Automatic Attending, and a General Theory. *Psychol Rev* 1977;84(2):127-190.

(26) Ariely D. Cash versus Credit. *http://danariely.com/2013/03/21/cash-versus-credit/*. 2013 March 21. Accessed March 31, 2014.

(27) Ariely D. Societe Generale - behavioral economics at work. *http://danariely.com/2008/02/01/societe-generale-%E2%80%93-behavioral-economics-at-work/.* 2008 February 1. Accessed March 31, 2014.

(28) Ariely D. Ask Ariely: On Tesla, To-Do Lists, and Knowing the News. *http://danariely.com/2013/10/14/ask-ariely-on-tesla-to-do-lists-and-knowing-the-news/.* 2013 October 14. Accessed October 15, 2013.

(29) Ariely D. The Pain of Paying: The Psychology of Money. *http://blogs.fuqua.duke.edu/facultyconversations/2013/01/14/dan-ariely/.* 2013 February. Accessed March 31, 2014.

(30) Thaler RH, Sunstein CR. *Nudge: Improving Decisions About Health, Wealth, and Happiness, Revised and Expanded Edition.* New York: Penguin; 2009.

(31) Loewenstein G, Asch DA, Volpp KG. Behavioral Economics Holds Potential To Deliver Better Results For Patients, Insurers, And Employers. *Health Aff (Millwood)* 2013;32(7):1244-1250.

(32) Tuong W, Armstrong AW. Effect of appearance-based education compared with health-based education on sunscreen use and knowledge: A randomized controlled trial. *J Am Acad Dermatol* 2014;70(4):665-669.

(33) Ariely D. *Predictably Irrational: The Hidden Forces that Shape Our Decisions.* New York: HarperCollins; 2008.

(34) Mochon D, Norton MI, Ariely D. Bolstering and Restoring Feelings of Competence via the IKEA Effect. *Int J Res Marketing* 2012;29(4):363-369.

(35) Allais M. Le comportement de l'homme rationnel devant le risque: Critique des postulats et axiomes de l'Ecole Americaine. *Econometrica* 1953;21:503-546.

(36) Benartzi S, Thaler RH. Heuristics and Biases in Retirement Savings Behavior. *J Econ Perspect* 2007;21(3):81-104.

(37) Thaler RH, Mullainathan S. Behavioral Economics. *http://www.econlib.org/library/Enc/BehavioralEconomics.html.* 2008. Accessed November 18, 2013.

(38) Madrian B, Shea D. The Power of Suggestion: Inertia in 401(k) Participation and Savings Behavior. *Q J Econ* 2001;116(4):1149-1187.

(39) Michielsen P. Presumed Consent to Organ Donation: 10 Years' Experience in Belgium. *J Royal Soc Med* 1996;89:663-666.

(40) Thaler RH. Toward a positive theory of consumer choice. *J Econ Behav Org* 1980;1:39-60.

(41) Thaler RH. Mental Accounting Matters. *J Behav Decision Making* 1999;12:183-206.

(42) Sindelar JL, O'Malley SS. Financial versus health motivation to quit smoking: A randomized field study. *Prev Med* 2013;(13):10.

(43) Huber J, Payne JW, Puto C. Adding Asymmetrically Dominated Alternatives: Violations of Regularity and the Similarity Hypothesis. *J Consumer Res* 1982;9(1):90-98.

(44) Russo JE, Rosen LD. An eye fixation analysis of multialternative choice. *Mem Cognit* 1975;3(3):267-276.

(45) Thorndike EL. A constant error in psychological ratings. *J Appl Psych* 1920;4(1):25-29.

(46) Sigall H, Ostrove N. Beautiful but Dangerous: Effects of Offender Attractiveness and Nature of the Crime on Juridic Judgment. *J Personal Soc Psychol* 1975;31(3):410-414.

(47) Uhas AA, Camacho FT, Feldman SR, Balkrishnan R. The Relationship Between Physician Friendliness and Caring, and Patient Satisfaction: Findings from an Internet-Based Survey. *Patient* 2008;1(2):91-96.

(48) Rajpara AN, Landis ET, Feldman SR. Office Evaluation: Gaining a Fresh Perspective. *http://www.the-dermatologist.com/content/office-evaluation-gaining-fresh-perspective*. 2012 May. Accessed October 4, 2013.

(49) Ariely D. Ask Ariely: On Dog Droppings, Working Late, and Trying Out Girlfriends. *http://danariely.com/2013/04/27/ask-ariely-on-dog-droppings-working-late-and-trying-out-girlfriends/.* 2013 April 27. Accessed October 25, 2013.

(50) Parks L, Balkrishnan R, Hamel-Gariepy L, Feldman SR. The importance of skin disease as assessed by "willingness-to-pay". *J Cutan Med Surg* 2003;7(5):369-371.

(51) American Society for Aesthetic Plastic Surgery. Is Botox recession-proof? *http://www.surgery.org/consumers/plastic-surgery-news-briefs/botox-recession-proof-1035592*. 2011 September 23. Accessed October 25, 2013.

(52) Camerer C, Loewenstein G, Weber M. The curse of knowledge in economic settings: An experimental analysis. *J Polit Econ* 1989;97:1232-1254.

(53) Newton L. Overconfidence in the communication of intent: Heard and unheard melodies. 1990.
Ref Type: Unpublished Work

(54) Heath C, Heath D. *Made to Stick: Why Some Ideas Survive and Others Die*. New York: Random House; 2007.

(55) Heath C, Heath D. Made to Stick SUCCESs Model. *http://heathbrothers.com/download/mts-made-to-stick-model.pdf*. 2008. Accessed April 8, 2014.

(56) Feldman SR. *Practical Ways to Improve Patients' Treatment Outcomes*. Winston-Salem: Medical Quality Enhancement Corporation; 2009.

(57) Milgram S. Behavioral Study of Obedience. *J Abnorm Soc Psychol* 1963;67(4):371-378.

(58) Asch SE. Opinions and social pressure. *Sci Am* 1955;193(5):31-35.

(59) Hertz N. Why We Make Bad Decisions. *http://www.nytimes.com/2013/10/20/opinion/sunday/why-we-make-bad-decisions.html?_r=0*. 2013 October 19. Accessed November 5, 2013.

(60) Feldman SR. *Compartments: How the Brightest, Best Trained, and Most Caring People can Make Judgments That are Completely and Utterly Wrong*. Xlibris; 2009.

(61) Dillard JP, Shen L. On the Nature of Reactance and its Role in Persuasive Health Communication. *Commun Monogr* 2005;72(2):144-168.

(62) Miller CH, Lane LT, Deatrick LM, Young AM, Potts KA. Psychological Reactance and Promotional Health Messages: The Effects of Controlling Language, Lexical Concreteness, and the Restoration of Freedom. *Hum Commun Res* 2007;33(2):219-240.

(63) Cole SA, Bird J. *The Medical Interview: The Three-Function Approach*. 2 ed. St. Louis: Mosby; 2000.

(64) Rollnick S, Butler CC, Kinnersley P, Gregory J, Mash B. Motivational interviewing. *BMJ* 2010;340:c1900. doi: 10.1136/bmj.c1900.:c1900.

(65) The Rudd Center for Food Policy and Obesity. Improving Patient-Provider Interactions: Motivational interviewing for diet/exercise and obesity. *http://www.yaleruddcenter.org/resources/bias_toolkit/toolkit/ Module-2/2-07-MotivationalStrategies.pdf*. 2011. Accessed November 5, 2013.

(66) Feldman S, Davis S. Practical implications of behavioral economics for dermatology practice. *https://www.dermquest.com/expert-opinions/opinions-on-practice-management/2013/practical-implications-of-behavioral-economics-for-dermatology-practice*. 2013 July 10. Accessed December 7, 2013.

(67) Miller WR, Rollnick S. *Motivational Interviewing: Preparing People to Change*. New York: Guilford; 2002.

(68) Channon S, Smith VJ, Gregory JW. A pilot study of motivational interviewing in adolescents with diabetes. *Arch Dis Child* 2003;88(8):680-683.

(69) Ryan RM, Deci EL. Intrinsic and Extrinsic Motivations: Classic Definitions and New Directions. *Contemp Educ Psychol* 2000;25(1):54-67.

(70) Delong M, Winter D. *Learning to Teach and Teaching to Learn Mathematics: Resources for Professional Development.* Mathematical Association of America; 2002.

(71) Dewinstanley PA, Bjork EL. Processing strategies and the generation effect. *Mem Cognit* 2004;32(6):945-955.

(72) Slamecka NJ, Graf P. The generation effect: delineation of a phenomenon. *J Exp Psychol* 1978;4:592-604.

(73) McMahon M. What is the Generation Effect? *http://www.wisegeek.com/what-is-the-generation-effect.htm.* 2013 March 15. Accessed January 8, 2014.

(74) Hackman JR, Lawler EE. Employee reaction to job characteristics. *J Appl Psych Monogr* 1971;55:259-286.

(75) Phillips JM, Gully SM. *Organizational behavior: Tools for success.* Mason, OH: Cengage Learning; 2012.

(76) Morgeson FP, Johnson MD, Campion MA, Medsker GJ, Mumford TV. Understanding Reactions to Job Redesign: A Quasi-Experimental Investigation of the Moderating Effects of Organizational Context on Perceptions of Performance Behavior. *Personnel Psychol* 2006;59:333-363.

(77) Grandpre J, Alvaro EM, Burgoon M, Miller CH, Hall JR. Adolescent reactance and anti-smoking campaigns: A theoretical approach. *Health Commun* 2003;15:349-366.

(78) Nevins TE. Non-compliance and its management in teenagers. *Pediatr Transplant* 2002;6(6):475-479.

(79) Yentzer BA, Gosnell AL, Clark AR et al. A randomized controlled pilot study of strategies to increase adherence in teenagers with acne vulgaris. *J Am Acad Dermatol* 2011;64(4):793-795.

(80) Boker A, Feetham HJ, Armstrong A, Purcell P, Jacobe H. Do automated text messages increase adherence to acne therapy? Results of a randomized, controlled trial. *J Am Acad Dermatol* 2012;67(6):1136-1142.

(81) Yentzer BA, Wood AA, Sagransky MJ et al. An internet-based survey and improvement of acne treatment outcomes. *Arch Dermatol* 2011;147(10):1223-1224.

(82) North Carolina Program on Health Literacy. The Teach-Back Method. *http://www.nchealthliteracy.org/toolkit/tool5.pdf.* 2014. Accessed January 13, 2014.

(83) Glovsky ER. Motivational Interviewing - Listening for Change Talk. *http://www.recoverytoday.net/archive/19-june/45-motivational-interviewing-listening-for-change-talk.* 2011. Accessed May 19, 2014.

(84) Sedgwick County Corrections. Motivational Interviewing Desk Reference. *http://www.sedgwickcounty.org/corrections/Motivational%20Interviewing/Motivational%20Interviewing%20Desk%20REFERENCE%20Guide.pdf.* 2014. Accessed May 19, 2014.

(85) Slovic P, Fischhoff B, Lichtenstein S. Response mode, framing, and information-processing effects in risk assessment. In: Hogarth R, editor. *New directions for methodology of social and behavioral science: Question framing and response consistency.* San Francisco: Jossey-Bass; 1982. 21-36.

(86) Novemsky N, Kahneman D. The Boundaries of Loss Aversion. *J Market Res* 2005;42:119-128.

(87) Carroll RT. Negativity Bias. *http://www.skepdic.com/negativitybias.html* 2014. Accessed January 22, 2014.

(88) Baumeister RF, Bratslavsky E, Finkenauer C, Vohs DK. Bad is Stronger than Good. *Rev Gen Psychol* 2001;5(4):323-370.

(89) Brickman P, Coates D, Janoff-Bulman R. Lottery winners and accident victims: Is happiness relative? *J Personal Soc Psychol* 1978;36:917-927.

(90) Rozin P, Royzman BE. Negativity Bias, Negativity Dominance, and Cognition. *Personal Soc Psychol Rev* 2001;5(4):296-320.

(91) Mizerski RW. An attribution explanation of the disproportionate influence of unfavorable information. *J Consumer Res* 1982;9(3):301-310.

(92) Richey MH, Koenigs RJ, Richey HW, Fortin R. Negative Salience in Impressions of Character: Effects of Unequal Proportions of Positive and Negative Information. *J Soc Psychol* 1975;97:233-241.

(93) Matos CA, Veiga RT. The Effects of Negative Publicity on Consumer Attitudes: a replication and extension. *http://papers.ssrn.com/sol3/papers.cfm?abstract_id=599281.* 2004. Accessed February 14, 2014.

(94) Kepplinger HM, Sonja G. Research Note: Reciprocal Effects of Negative Press Reports. *Eur J Commun* 2007;22:337-354.

(95) Hanson R. Confronting the Negativity Bias. *http://www.huffingtonpost.com/rick-hanson-phd/be-mindful-not-intimidate_b_753646.html*. 2010 October 8. Accessed January 24, 2014.

(96) Griffin M, Babin BJ, Attaway JS. An Empirical Investigation of the Impact of Negative Public Publicity on Consumer Attitudes and Intentions. *Adv Consum Res* 1991;18:334-341.

(97) Travaline JM, Ruchinskas R, D'Alonzo GE, Jr. Patient-Physician Communication: Why and How. *J Am Osteopath Assoc* 2005;105(1):13-18.

(98) Roter DL, Frankel MR, Hall JA, Sluyter D. The Expression of Emotion Through Nonverbal Behavior in Medical Visits: Mechanisms and Outcomes. *J Gen Intern Med* 2006;21(1):28-34.

(99) Milmoe S, Rosenthal R, Blane HT, Chafetz ME, Wolf I. The doctor's voice: postdictor of successful referral of alcoholic patients. *J Abn Psychol* 1967;72:78-84.

(100) Coombs CH, Bezembinder TG, Goode FM. Testing Expectation Theories of Decision Making without Measuring Utility or Subjective Probability. *J Math Psychol* 1967;4:72-103.

(101) Carmon Z, Ariely D. Focusing on the forgone: How value can appear so different to buyers and sellers. *J Consumer Res* 2000;27:360-370.

(102) Gladwell M. *Outliers: The Story of Success*. New York: Little, Brown, and Company; 2008.

(103) Ariely D, Kamenica E, Prelec D. Man's search for meaning: The case of Legos. *J Econ Behav Org* 2008;67:671-677.

(104) Rogers T, Fox CR, Gerber AS. Rethinking Why People Vote: Voting as Dynamic Social Expression. In: Shafir E, editor. *The Behavioral Foundations of Public Policy*.Princeton: Princeton UP; 2013.

(105) Carnegie D. *How to Win Friends and Influence People.* New York: Simon & Schuster; 1981.

(106) World Health Organization. Adherence to long-term therapies: evidence for action. *http://apps.who.int/medicinedocs/pdf/s4883e/s4883e.pdf.* 2003. Accessed January 4, 2014.

(107) Haisley E, Volpp KG, Pellathy T, Loewenstein G. The impact of alternative incentive schemes on completion of health risk assessments. *Am J Health Promot* 2012;26(3):184-188.

(108) Baum S. Are charity donations the key to medication adherence? Janssen tests that theory with medication reminder app. *http://medcitynews.com/2013/09/charity-donations-key-medication-adherence-janssens-tests-theory-medication-reminder-app/.* 2013 September. Accessed January 15, 2014.

(109) Kelley D, Kelley T. *Creative Confidence: Unleashing the Creative Potential within Us All.* Crown Business; 2013.

(110) Evans JS, Barston JL, Pollard P. On the conflict between logic and belief in syllogistic reasoning. *Mem Cognit* 1983;11(3):295-306.

(111) Newstead SE, Pollard P, Evans JS, Allen JL. The source of belief bias effects in syllogistic reasoning. *Cognition* 1992;45(3):257-284.

(112) Sa WC, West RF, Stanovich KE. The domain specificity and generality of belief bias. *J Educ Psychol* 1999;91(3):497-510.

(113) Morley NJ, Evans JS, Handley SJ. Belief bias and figural bias in syllogistic reasoning. *Q J Exp Psychol A* 2004;57(4):666-692.

(114) Cooper RA, Jenkins L. A Comparison Between Medical Grade Honey and Table Honeys in Relation to Antimicrobial Efficacy. *Wounds* 2009;21(2):29-36.

(115) Sternberg RJ, Leighton JP. *The Nature of Reasoning.* New York: Cambridge UP; 2004.

(116) Markovits H, Nantel G. The belief-bias effect in the production and evaluation of logical conclusions. *Mem Cognit* 1989;17(1):11-17.

(117) Diener E, Lucas RE, Scollon CN. Beyond the hedonic treadmill: revising the adaptation theory of well-being. *Am Psychologist* 2006;61(4):305-314.

(118) Brickman P, Campbell DT. Hedonic relativism and planning the good society. In: Appley MH, editor. *Adaption Level Theory: A Symposium.*New York: Academic Press; 1971. 287-302.

(119) Suh E, Diener E, Fujita F. Events and subjective well-being: Only recent events matter. *J Personal Soc Psychol* 1996;70:1091-1102.

(120) Taylor SE, Lichtman RR, Wood JV. Attributions, beliefs about control, and adjustment to breast cancer. *J Pers Soc Psychol* 1984;46(3):489-502.

(121) Feinman S. The Blind as 'Ordinary People'. *J Vis Impair Blind* 1978;72:231-238.

(122) Silver RL. Coping with an undesirable life event: A study of early reactions to physical disability. Northwestern University; 1982.

(123) Nolan BV, Feldman SR. Adherence, the fourth dimension in the geometry of dermatological treatment. *Arch Dermatol* 2009;145(11):1319-1321.

(124) Ali SM, Brodell RT, Balkrishnan R, Feldman SR. Poor adherence to treatments: a fundamental principle of dermatology. *Arch Dermatol* 2007;143(7):912-915.

(125) Davis SA, Feldman SR. Practical Implications of Behavioral Economics for Dermatology Practice: Part 2. *https://www.dermquest.com/expert-opinions/opinions-on-practice-management/2013/practical-implications-of-behavioral-economics-for-dermatology-practice-part-2*. 2013 November 20. Accessed April 17, 2014.

(126) Easterlin RA. Does Economic Growth Improve the Human Lot? Some Empirical Evidence. In: David PA, Reder MW, editors. *Nations and Households in Economic Growth: Essays in Honor of Moses Abramovitz.*New York: Academic Press; 1974.

(127) Cantril H. *The Pattern of Human Concerns.* New Brunswick, NJ: Rutgers UP; 1965.

(128) Dunn E, Norton M. *Happy Money: The Science of Smarter Spending.* New York: Simon & Schuster; 2013.

(129)   Balboni T, Balboni M, Paulk ME et al. Support of cancer patients' spiritual needs and associations with medical care costs at the end of life. *Cancer* 2011;117(23):5383-5391.

(130)   Galai D, Sade O. The 'Ostrich Effect' and the Relationship between the Liquidity and the Yields of Financial Assets. *http://papers.ssrn.com/sol3/papers.cfm?abstract_id=431180*. 2003 July. Accessed November 11, 2013.

(131)   Karlsson N, Loewenstein G, Seppi D. The ostrich effect: Selective attention to information. *J Risk Uncertain* 2009;38:95-115.

(132)   Weeks AL. *Stalin's Other War: Soviet Grand Strategy, 1939-1941*. Rowman & Littlefield; 2003.

(133)   Sorscher S. Group-think Caused the Market to Fail. *http://www.huffingtonpost.com/stan-sorscher/group-think-caused-the-ma_b_604810.html*. 2010 June 9. Accessed November 12, 2013.

(134)   Investopedia. Ostrich Definition. *http://www.investopedia.com/terms/o/ostrich.asp*. 2013. Accessed November 11, 2013.

(135)   Lund-Nielsen B, Midtgaard J, Rorth M, Gottrup F, Adamsen L. An avalanche of ignoring--a qualitative study of health care avoidance in women with malignant breast cancer wounds. *Cancer Nurs* 2011;34(4):277-285.

(136)   Davis SA, Feldman SR. Using Hawthorne Effects to Improve Adherence in Clinical Practice: Lessons from Clinical Trials. *JAMA Dermatol* 2013;149(4):490-491.

(137) Mega Millions. How to Play. *http://www.megamillions.com/how-to-play*. 2013. Accessed December 19, 2013.

(138) Attneave F. Psychological probability as a function of increased frequency. *J Exp Psychol* 1953;46(2):81-86.

(139) Rottenstreich Y, Hsee CK. Money, Kisses, and Electric Shocks: On the Affective Psychology of Risk. *Psychol Sci* 2001;12(3):185-190.

(140) Camerer CF. Recent Tests of Generalizations of Expected Utility Theory. *Utility theories: measurements and applications.*Boston: Kluwer Academic Publishers; 1992. 207-251.

(141) Sunstein CR. Probability Neglect: Emotions, Worst Cases, and Law. *Yale Law J* 2002;112:61-107.

(142) Kunreuther H, Novemsky N, Kahneman D. Making Low Probabilities Useful. *J Risk Uncertain* 2001;23(2):103-120.

(143) Baron J. *Thinking and Deciding*. 3 ed. Cambridge, England: Cambridge UP; 2000.

(144) Haisley E, Mostafa R, Loewenstein G. Subjective Relative Income and Lottery Ticket Purchases. *J Behav Dec Making* 2008;21:283-295.

(145) Mischel W, Ebbesen EB. Attention in delay of gratification. *J Pers Soc Psychol* 1970;16(2):329-337.

(146) Mischel W, Ebbesen EB, Zeiss AR. Cognitive and attentional mechanisms in delay of gratification. *J Pers Soc Psychol* 1972;21(2):204-218.

(147) Danziger S, Levav J, Avnaim-Pesso L. Extraneous factors in judicial decisions. *Proc Natl Acad Sci U S A* 2011;108(17):6889-6892.

(148) Gailliot MT, Baumeister RF, DeWall CN et al. Self-control relies on glucose as a limited energy source: willpower is more than a metaphor. *J Pers Soc Psychol* 2007;92(2):325-336.

(149) Baumeister RF. Self-control: the moral muscle. *Psychologist* 2012;25(2):12-15.

(150) Baer D. Always Wear the Same Suit: Obama's Presidential Productivity Secrets. *http://www.fastcompany.com/3026265/work-smart/always-wear-the-same-suit-obamas-presidential-productivity-secrets.* 2014 February 12. Accessed March 4, 2014.

(151) Rice T. The behavioral economics of health and health care. *Annu Rev Public Health* 2013;34:431-47. doi: 10.1146/annurev-publhealth-031912-114353. Epub;%2013 Jan 7.:431-447.

(152) Wansink B, van IK. Portion size me: plate-size induced consumption norms and win-win solutions for reducing food intake and waste. *J Exp Psychol Appl* 2013;19(4):320-332.

(153) Thorgeirsson T, Kawachi I. Behavioral economics: merging psychology and economics for lifestyle interventions. *Am J Prev Med* 2013;44(2):185-189.

(154) Wansink B, van IK. Shape of glass and amount of alcohol poured: comparative study of effect of practice and concentration. *BMJ* 2005;331(7531):1512-1514.

(155) Norman D. Nutrition, Nudges, and Sledge Hammers. *http://www.linkedin.com/today/post/article/20140301024625 -12181762-nutrition-nudges-and-sledge-hammers.* 2014 March 1. Accessed March 4, 2014.

(156) Steiner JF, Robbins LJ, Roth SC, Hammond WS. The effect of prescription size on acquisition of maintenance medications. *J Gen Intern Med* 1993;8(6):306-310.

(157) Coombs JH, Cornish L, Hiller P, Smith DG. Compliance and refill pattern behavior with HMG-CoA reductase inhibitors after acute myocardial infarction. *Manag Care Interface* 2002;15(1):54-8, 60.

(158) Laibson D. Golden eggs and hyperbolic discounting. *Q J Econ* 1997;443-477.

(159) Strotz RH. Myopia and inconsistency in dynamic utility maximization. *Rev Econ Stud* 1956;23:165-180.

(160) Stein KB, Sarbin TR, Kulik JA. Future time perspective: Its relation to the socialization process and the delinquent role. *J Consult Clin Psychol* 1968;32:257-264.

(161) Freud S. Formulations on the two principles of mental functioning. In: Strachey J, Freud A, editors. *The standard edition of the complete psychological works of Sigmund Freud.*London: Hogarth; 1956.

(162) Hartman H. Notes on the reality principle. *Psychoanal Stud Chil* 1956;11:31-53.

(163) Killeen P. Preference for fixed-interval schedules of reinforcement. *J Exp Anal Behav* 1970;14:127-131.

(164) Mowrer OH, Ullman AD. Time as a determinant in integrative learning. *Psychol Rev* 1945;52:61-90.

(165) Kanfer FH, Phillips J. *Learning foundations of behavior therapy*. New York: Wiley; 1970.

(166) Akerlof GA, Dickens WF. The economic consequences of cognitive dissonance. *Am Econ Rev* 1982;72:307-319.

(167) Vuchinich RE, Simpson CA. Hyperbolic temporal discounting in social drinkers and problem drinkers. *Exp Clin Psychopharmacol* 1998;25:6-25.

(168) Mitchell S. Measures of impulsivity in cigarette smokers and non-smokers. *Psychopharmacology* 1999.

(169) Bickel WK, Odum AL, Madden GJ. Impulsivity and cigarette smoking: Delay discounting in current, never, and ex-smokers. *Psychopharmacology* 1999;146:447-454.

(170) Kirby KN, Petry NM, Bickel WK. Heroin addicts have higher discount rates for delayed rewards than non-drug-using controls. *J Exp Psychol* 1999;128:78-87.

(171) Wallace C. The effects of delayed rewards, social pressure, and frustration on the response of opiate addicts. *NIDA Monograph Series* 1979;25:6-25.

(172) Monterosso J, Ainslie G. The behavioral economics of will in recovery from addiction. *Drug Alcohol Depend* 2007;90:S100-S111.

(173) Aristotle. *The complete works of Aristotle*. Princeton: Princeton UP; 1984.

(174) Kirby KN, Guastello B. Making choices in anticipation of similar future choices can increase self-control. *J Exp Psychol* 2001;7:154-164.

(175) Mitchell TR, Thompson L, Peterson E, Cronk R. Temporal adjustments in the evaluation of events: The "rosy view". *J Exp Soc Psychol* 1997;33:421-448.

(176) Klaaren KJ, Hodges SD, Wilson TD. The role of affective expectations in subjective experience and decision making. *Soc Cognit* 1994;12:77-101.

(177) Ariely D, Carmon Z. Summary Assessment of Experiences: The Whole is different from the Sum of its Parts. *http://web.mit.edu/ariely/www/MIT/Chapters/seqC.pdf.* 2013. Accessed December 2, 2013.

(178) Saffrey C, Summerville A, Roese NJ. Praise for regret: People value regret above other negative emotions. *Motiv Emot* 2008;32(1):46-54.

(179) Gilbert DT, Morewedge CK, Risen JL, Wilson TD. Looking Forward to Looking Backward: The Misprediction of Regret. *Psychol Sci* 2004;15(5):346-350.

(180) Ariely D. Dear Irrational (is it rational to visit mother?). *http://danariely.com/2008/04/19/dear-irrational-is-it-rational-to-visit-mother/.* 2008 April 19. Accessed December 31, 2013.

(181) Ariely D. Admitting to another irrationality. *http://danariely.com/2011/03/10/admitting-to-another-irrationality/.* 2011 March 10. Accessed December 31, 2013.

(182) Ariely D. Ask Ariely: On the Lottery, Corporate Charity, and Maternalism. *http://danariely.com/2013/10/26/ask-ariely-on-the-lottery-corporate-charity-and-maternalism/.* 2013 October 26. Accessed December 31, 2013.

(183) Sandberg T, Conner M. A mere measurement effect for anticipated regret: Impacts on cervical screening attendance. *Br J Soc Psychol* 2009;48:221-236.

(184) O'Carroll RE, Dryden J, Hamilton-Barclay T, Ferguson E. Anticipated regret and organ donor registration--a pilot study. *Health Psychol* 2011;30(5):661-664.

(185) Shepherd L, O'Carroll R. When do Next-of-Kin Opt-In? Anticipated Regret, Affective Attitudes and Donating Deceased Family Member's Organs. *J Health Psychol* 2013.

(186) Medvec VH, Madey SF, Gilovich T. When less is more: counterfactual thinking and satisfaction among Olympic medalists. *J Pers Soc Psychol* 1995;69(4):603-610.

(187) Sarwer DB. The "obsessive" cosmetic surgery patient: a consideration of body image dissatisfaction and body dysmorphic disorder. *Plast Surg Nurs* 1997;17(4):193-197.

(188) Ariely D, Wertenbroch K. Procrastination, deadlines, and performance: Self-control by precommitment. *Psychol Sci* 2002;13(3):219-224.

(189) Thaler RH, Benartzi S. Save more tomorrow(TM): Using behavioral economics to increase employee saving. *J Polit Econ* 2004;112(S1):S164-S187.

(190) Ariely D. Procrastination. *http://danariely.com/tag/procrastination/.* 2009 November 15. Accessed February 2, 2014.

Scott A. Davis, MA, is Assistant Director of the Center for Dermatology Research at Wake Forest School of Medicine. He won first prize in the Poster Walk at the 2011 European Society for Patient Adherence, Compliance, and Persistence (ESPACOMP) meeting in Utrecht, Netherlands for research on an Internet-based survey to improve acne adherence. In fall 2014 he will begin PhD studies as a Royster Fellow at the UNC Eshelman School of Pharmacy, in Pharmaceutical Outcomes and Policy. His research focuses on health care delivery and interventions to improve adherence to healthy behaviors. He graduated from the University of Chicago.

Steven R. Feldman, MD, PhD, is Professor of Dermatology, Pathology, and Public Health Sciences at Wake Forest School of Medicine, and Director of the Center for Dermatology Research, a health services research center funded by a grant from Galderma Laboratories, L.P. He received a Presidential Citation from the American Academy of Dermatology in 2005 for his psoriasis education efforts and received one of the AAD's highest awards, the Clarence S. Livingood Lectureship, at the 2006 AAD Meeting. His research studies into patients' adherence to their topical treatments helped transform how dermatologists understand and manipulate patients' use of topical medications over the course of chronic disease. Dr. Feldman was awarded an Astellas Award by the American Academy of Dermatology in 2008 for scientific research that has improved public health in the field of dermatology. He is also the founder of Medical Quality Enhancement Corporation, DrScore.com, and Causa Research. His 15 other books include *Compartments: How the Brightest, Best Trained, and Most Caring People can make Judgments That are Completely & Utterly Wrong.*

Made in the USA
Charleston, SC
16 June 2014